# The Health and Medical Use of
# *Aloe Vera*

Dr. Lawrence G. Plaskett

Life Sciences Press
Tacoma, WA

Library of Congress Cataloging-in-Publication Data

Plaskett, L.G.
The health amd medical use of aloe vera / Lawrence G. Plaskett.
p.  cm.
Includes bibliographical references.
Indexed


ISBN 0-943685-21-4


1. Aloe barbadensis--Therapeutic use.  I. Title
RM666.A414P56   1996
615'.324324--dc20                                          96-32704
                                                           CIP

cover photo

The presence of the brass tap and collecting vessel is a
humorous representation of the collection of Aloe exudate: in
practice the yellowish exudate runs freely from the cut ends of
the leaves.

# The Health & Medical Use of
# *Aloe vera*

## *CONTENTS*

# Foreword

Welcome to a new world vision for *Aloe vera*. *Aloe vera* has been used for thousands of years and is today American's #1 home remedy. In fact, Aloe vera is one of the best natural products for the healthful benefit of mankind. The Aloe industry is moving towards a higher standard of excel-lence in product quality and purity. Correct and thoroughly researched information fuels this drive for excellence. I believe in and am pleased to be a part of this growing tradition of excellence. It is an honor to be associated with the depth of information represented in Dr. Plaskett's book.

As the industry continues to devote itself to quality processing, recognized standards of purity, unbiased information, truth in labeling and shared results of scientific discovery the entire world will benefit from Nature's Miracle Plant. The miracle of the plant itself demands the best possible effort from everyone involved in the industry. I encourage all who learn from Dr. Plaskett's book to take the high road of *Aloe vera* excellence. Set your sights on purity and honesty and know that mankind will receive a 'cascade' of medical benefit.

With this book, Dr. Plaskett accomplishes the major task of outlining the various biological activities of Aloe vera with a synopsis of past scientific research. Dr. Plaskett is paving the way for research and analysis to carefully catalog exactly how *Aloe vera* works in the human body. This book helps us better understand Aloe's biologically active components. Thank you Dr. Plaskett.

L. Scott McKnight
President, Aloe Commodities International, Inc.
Founder, International Aloe Science Council

i

# Dr. Lawrence G. Plaskett

Lawrence graduated from Cambridge in Natural Sciences, specializing in biochemistry. He then did medical research on thyroid hormones with the Medical Research Council, obtaining his doctorate. For five years he become a Lecturer in Biochemistry at Edinburgh University Medical School and his research enlarged the knowledge then available about T3, the principal thyroid hormone.

He then worked as Corporate Research Director of the Brook Bond Liebig Group. His department was responsible for the development of food and food ingredient products for the Group world-wide. He conducted innovative research into novel protein foods, instant tea manufacture, essential oils, ad oleoresins as well as general food product formulations. During this time he became a Chartered Chemist and a Fellow of the Royal Society of Chemistry (C.Chem. FRSC) and a Fellow of the Institute of Food Science and Technology (FIFST).

In this role he became responsible for a major technical and agronomic program to diversify the business activities of the Group's tea and coffee plantations and ranch lands, in all amounting to some 1,100,000 acres worldwide, and became involved in producing a number of medicinally important substances from plantation crops. From that point onward Lawrence has maintained an intense interest in economically and medically important biochemicals produced from plants and optimizing their production and use, including the extraction technology required for these special compounds, as well as the biochemistry of their structure and their synthesis within the plant. The whole subject of pharmacognosy (medicines from plants) therefore became an absorbing life-time interest, addressing many questions of how the enormous diversity of plant biochemistry can be best harnessed to human advantage. These days he applies this interest especially to the field of natural products and health products. He now acts as consultant to a number of companies in this field.

He established his own Biotechnology Consultancy and Process Development Company serving the Food and Energy Industries working for many public companies and governmental or intergovernmental agencies  He also established a company for the sale of high quality vitamin and mineral products of his own concept and design. Today, however, he concentrates upon writing, research, and training practitioners of nutritional medicine.

His principle aim now is to make a progressively more profound synthesis of comprehension between nutrition and metabolism on the one hand, and the incidence of medical pathology on the other. He sees modern biochemistry being the basis of a very important bridge that can be built relating the causes of medical conditions to the underlying cellular biochemistry. He is personally able to embrace these fields by dint of his own personal philosophy of medicine and his life-long experience working in the borderlands between nutrition and medicine, in which he synthesizes the many interrelated disciplines into a coherent whole. Against this background, his work on Aloe has been a penetrating inquiry, the results and conclusions from which are presented in this book.

# AUTHOR'S PREFACE

There are already many books on *Aloe vera* - the wonder medicine plant. Mostly they are books written by out and out enthusiasts for this renowned herbal remedy. In answer to the obvious question, "why do we need another book on *Aloe vera* ?" I have no hesitation in saying that this author writes from the standpoint of an investigator rather than that of an out and out enthusiast. Whilst willingly admitting that this is a field in which most investigators seem to end up as enthusiasts (a fact which must illustrate something!), I do believe that I have succeeded in maintaining an investigator's objectivity throughout my inquire. Most people who have written books about Aloe are not scientists, and certainly are not senior scientists with forty or more years of experience of investigations to their credit in the borderlands between nutrition and medicine.

At the very core of the raison d'être for the book lies a determination to find out what science and scientific medicine really know about Aloe. There are many topics within herbal medicine and among the concepts of alternative or complementary medicine which are almost untouched by the hand of science. Often these may just not have attracted the attentions of research scientists, or, perhaps they are topics which are simply not "respectable" for self respecting scientists to investigate. Sometimes a scientist finds himself or herself in a post wherein, to turn any professional attention to a topic which smacks of the alternative or complementary, would amount to a heresy which would be more than their job is worth. Many intriguing topics are excluded in this manner from the range of subjects covered within the world of the medical sciences. Would Aloe be one of these? Would I find a dearth of information about Aloe in the respected scientific journals? The more than delicate subject of funding comes in here also. Research always costs money and who would fund research which would never earn very much money for the pharmaceutical companies?

In the particular instance of Aloe I need not have worried. Scientists and occasionally doctors around the world had shown a sporadic interest in Aloe which led them into producing the odd once-off paper in the journals. They could be from India, Kuwait, Egypt, China or the Ukraine. Often the author or group of authors would appear upon the Aloe scene with one or two published papers and then disappear from view. Nonetheless the accumulated significance of work from such authors could be considerable. Another type of publication arose specifically from Japan where investigators started to produce a spate of published papers from the late 1960's onwards, mainly from two centers of excellence. Clearly, Aloe was of practical importance medically in Japan, even though it was not mainly *Aloe vera* which they used, and some people there were determined to get to the bottom of the problem of

iii

just why it worked. The third group were the American researchers, especially those receiving serious funding from the Aloe industry itself, and these became increasingly significant through the 1980's and even more so in the 1990's. I found this an entirely favorable development. Admittedly, Aloe was originally being marketed in the USA on the basis of its mysterious, though impressive reputation and upon faith, imagination and, often, a considerable amount of hype. The fact that people believed in it and bought it led to the industry having a certain amount of financial muscle to a degree not often encountered in companies which serve the alternative and complementary field. The industry had "come of age" to the point where there was at least a modest surplus that could be spent upon technical improvements and, most particularly, upon finding out why the product worked. Moreover, all their work would be specifically with *Aloe vera*.

I found an amazing number of research papers from these three sources that were contributing different information about Aloe. Altogether they were running into a few hundred. A large number of other articles were also appearing which reported upon Aloe in an anecdotal way - these were, in other words, non-scientific reports. That did not make them wrong, indeed, there were enough of them to make me feel that most of them had to be right. However, they were not the core of what I was looking for. My key question was "how much evidence is there which arises from mainstream scientific research which proves or explains, or which tends to prove or explain, the beneficial properties of Aloe in medical situations and for the maintenance of health?" The answer was "a great deal". If that was the case then why, for heavens sake, had it not been brought forward for the serious attention of medical practitioners world-wide?

Aloe has been shown to exert at least three key actions upon cells of the animal and human body which makes it a potent medicine that can vie with or excel some of the most potent drugs in the medical pharmacopoeia. Indeed, it combines its actions in such a way that no known drug can match. The combination of effects makes it unique. At the same time, in the forms commonly marketed, it is totally non-toxic and free from side effects. It leaves absolutely no poisonous residues within the body after its use. Moreover, it stimulates the body to cleanse itself in an active, positive way that no known drug can mimic. That is not what the scientific papers say. But it is what I, as a biomedical scientist of 40 odd years of experience derive from what the scientific papers say.

Therefore, in this book I come to the intelligent, investigating, public, to the alternative and complementary practitioners and to the orthodox medical doctors to say as follows. "Look - here is the scientific literature on Aloe - much of it has existed for a decade or more and it is continuously growing. I have researched it, sifted it and interpreted it. This is what it means and this is my explanation of why it means what it does. If you are a holistically minded person - or perhaps a holistic practitioner - then I have both feet in your camp because I am one also. But my roots are in biomedical science. If

iv

you are orthodox, then I started out with both my feet in your camp". Here I am doing my best to bring together some of the threads of these two fields. To the holistically minded non-scientists I can say "Here, why not look at this science - it has something real to say - it has investigated this subject of Aloe with a rigor which holism and the Alternatives do not have. It has succeeded in proving something which you believed in anyway. Now you can believe in it even more. Probably it can achieve more than even you thought it would be able to do." Again to the orthodox I can say "this is your very own orthodox science yet it has proved in this case that something about an aspect of herbal medicine - something you have been doubtful about - is very, very right - probably more right than you ever thought possible. That may be frightening because it is outside the orthodox medical training - something which has nothing to do with pharmaceutical companies or operating theaters - but it calls for your urgent attention - most seriously so. It does not call upon you to believe in mysterious energies or philosophical systems which are outside the comprehension of science - this is fully comprehensible within science itself. Indeed, it is your very own orthodox science which in this case has proved out what you never expected it to prove - that this long renowned herb could be the most potent tool in your own armory of weapons against disease."

To the holistically minded I will say again - "no, I have not left the orthodox behind only to rejoin it again. I do consider that my search has substantially proved the case for *Aloe vera* in a manner which should be comprehensible to the orthodox, but that is only the tip of an iceberg. I am a senior scientist of long experience. I believe in leaving to science all that for which Science is ideally suited. But beware of ever becoming a slave to scientifically acquired knowledge. I know that you most probably never would have done so anyway. As a senior scientist I believe with you in the efficacy of homeopathic medicines, in the Chinese officials, in Prana and Chi, in the Chakras, in the energy meridians of acupuncture, in the powers of meditation and in the most subtle energies at work within Radionics. As a scientist I absolutely do not believe in science as the be-all and end-all of knowledge. A great many of us human beings have - in a historical sense - only just learned that Science is a useful and reliable way in which to acquire certain types of knowledge. The greater lesson which must inevitably follow after that is that what science can teach is only the very tip of a giant iceberg of knowledge. That science can only teach us about the grosser laws of matter and the grosser energies in the universe. All the rest, so far as science is concerned - still has to be appreciated, let alone learned. The conclusion: - science is, indeed, a most useful way to acquire knowledge - but only limitation and frustration can follow if one allows oneself to be cajoled into believing that science is the only, or even the principle, source from which human knowledge can flow."

This book started out as a scientific appraisal of Aloe. I think that is what it is. It provides scientific revelation and/or reassurance, if needed, to the effect that Aloe is a most potent medicine. This sort of scientific appraisal can, indeed, sometimes save the over-enthusiastic holist from going off at a tangent and being misled, perhaps, by his imagination. "Feet on the ground some of the time" is not a bad rule. If this book succeeds in convincing some people to use Aloe who would otherwise not have done so, that will be a good outcome, though it was not the original objective - which was just to investigate. The investigation has had a positive outcome and I am glad that this is so.

Alternative medicine may well benefit from having scientific validation some of the time. The last thing which I personally want anyone to believe is that I think there is any absolute necessity for it to have that validation. The higher insights of holism and of holistic medicine came from higher sources than the medical sciences of physiology and biochemistry. Therefore, if this little book is based upon science, then for me, it is science in the service of the higher energies - science in the service of naturopathy - and not the other way around.

*INTRODUCTION*

# THE NATURE OF THE PLANT AND ITS BACKGROUND

## Aloe - The Plant and its Relatives

The name "Aloe" applies to about 360 different species of related plants world-wide. They are related to each other by similarities of structure which have led botanists to classify them into their own group, or "genus" to which the Latin name given is "Aloe", the same as the name in colloquial use. This genus *Aloe* is a subdivision of the Lily Family, known as the "Liliaceae". Therefore, the plant has many relatives (i.e. within the same family) in Britain and still more in the United States. These include Lily-of-the-Valley, Star-of-Bethlehem, Bluebell, Asparagus, Onion, Leek, Grape Hyacinth, Garlic. Some of these share with Aloe the suitability for medical use. This is especially true of onion and garlic, the latter being widely used, of course, in the form of oils, extracts, capsules and tablets, while Star-of-Bethlehem is among the plants which contribute to the much renowned Bach flower remedies. None of these resemble Aloe at all, however, in appearance, because the above examples are all soft herbs, while the Aloes have a succulent character which suits them for survival in dry hot climates. This has led them to develop a rather tough impervious outer coat, the leaves being fibrous and strong. Their leaves contain a special type of tissue, which is adapted for moisture retention, comprising very large cells with very high water content amongst an ample supply of plant mucilage which has the property of binding large amounts of water. Their generally curved leaves characteristically develop spines at the edges, making them a particularly inhospitable type of vegetation amongst which to fall. They share some of these characteristics with

1

cacti, to which they are not related. The attachment positions of these are very closely packed on the stem, forming a dense rosette of tough spiky leaves as shown in Figures 1 and 2. At intervals the plants send up a flowering inflorescence on a long stem. To have plants in the same Family which look totally unlike each other is by no means unusual. The plant families have been classified according to the structure of their flowers and fruits rather than their gross appearance. These are considered by botanists to be the most fundamental aspects of plant structure, with aspects like size, toughness, appearance and climatic preferences being of lesser significance. This view embodies the belief that the Family evolved first, and then produced altered forms to adapt them to widely different habitats and environments, giving rise to multiple species.

## Aloes which are suited to medical use

Some of these Aloe plants have been considered to possess medical properties for a very long time, but this is limited to just a few species (i.e. individual members of the genus). The species are named by adding a second, species, name to the genus name "Aloe". The species which is most in evidence in Britain and the United States is generally being referred colloquially and commercially as *Aloe vera* but there continues to be some apparent disagreement or uncertainty about the true botanical, or official, name. The custom of botanists is to add to the official name an abbreviation of the surname of the botanist who discovered or first fully described the species. According to one view, the correct name is, indeed, *Aloe vera*, but to write it out in full it has to be *Aloe vera* (L.) Burm. f. On the other hand, the name *Aloe barbadensis* Miller appears to be much the most used name in scientific circles.

This ambiguity about the name is unfortunate, even more so because still other names have also been applied in the past and remain in the literature. These will be omitted here to avoid too much confusion. The other species which have been or are used include *Aloe ferox* Miller (Cape Aloes) and *Aloe perryi* Baker(Socotrine Aloes), whilst in the Far East, especially China and Japan, use is made of *Aloe arborensis* Miller and *Aloe saponaria*(Ait.) Haw. It seems clear from the numerous scientific reports on these plants that they all share some of the medicinal properties of *Aloe vera*, but there are most likely to be some important differences, which usually cannot be stated or quantified because most of the reported work has used only one species, offering no comparison with other species.

## The task of explaining Aloe's medical actions

The task of explaining the medicinal actions of Aloe is complex and difficult. In order to build up anything like a cohesive picture of how Aloe probably works, it is necessary to call upon all the available significant findings. It is necessary, therefore, to look at work that has been done whatever the species, and to try to draw up a picture of the mode of action using this work *across the board*. In particular, so much work has been done by Japanese scientists, using only *Aloe arborensis* and *Aloe saponaria*, that to ignore their work would entail foregoing some of the most inquiring and penetrating work in the field. The best policy, therefore, is to pool all this information regardless of species, though never forgetting that some conclusions could perhaps be flawed, so far as applying it to *Aloe vera* is concerned, because of species differences. On the whole, because one is studying different species of the same genus, it seems most probable that the biochemical similarities between them will be considerable. It is, perhaps, relatively unlikely that different species of Aloe will exert the same medical effect by completely different routes, though this is not impossible. It seems more likely that they will generally tend to share the same biochemical pathways to the same class of substances. They are more likely to differ in the relative amounts of these different substances which they produce, and therefore the predominating medical actions of this group of plants are likely to be available in different proportions and ratios from one species to another. Scientific readers will want to insist upon checking every finding in all the species of interest and comparing their potency in each particular effect. They are, of course, absolutely correct in this, given unlimited research funds to apply to Aloes, but it is not an ideal world; the amount of available scientific work is considerable and impressive but not unlimited. The intention here, therefore, is to use it all, wherever it relates to the information and understanding which one needs to create a synthesis of this information so as to produce an understandable picture of just how Aloe probably exerts its medical actions, and to consider the possibility of errors afterwards. The chances are, when looking in this way at closely related species, that one may, indeed, succeed in creating much understanding and making only a few minor mistakes which will have to be uncovered by further research. The author is very much in favor of this manner of treating scientific data and, apart from the understanding it generates, it tends to show clearly which categories of information most need checking out.

## The older history of the medical use of Aloe

Turning now to the medical actions that are ascribed to Aloes, it becomes immediately clear, that the origins of the medical uses are extremely ancient. Perhaps the very earliest reference is on 1700BC Sumarian Clay Tablets, in the World's oldest civilization located at the confluence of the rivers Tigris and Euphrates. The next is the Egyptian reference is to Egypt's "Papyrus Embers" in 1500BC. This is not surprising at all because Sumaria traded quite a lot with Egypt. The view of botanists generally is that the plant Aloe vera originated in the northern part of the African continent and that its use and cultivation spread out from there to many other parts of the World with suitable climate. If so the Aloes in Sumaria must have come originally from Africa. Perhaps, then, the Egyptians were after all the first users; there is a suggestion that an inscription on Egyptian tombs of around 4000BC actually refers to Aloes.

*Aloe vera* was used medicinally in Persia in ancient times and also used in the ancient Indian civilization and is still used in India today for its 1) cathartic, 2) stomachic, 3) emmenagogic and 4) antihelmitic properties. These terms mean, respectively, the same thing as 1) a laxative, 2) a medicine to improve stomach function, 3) a promoter of menstrual flow and 4) a worming preparation. Aloe has been an important medicine in China for centuries and it is still a common household remedy today. Specifically, *Aloe arborensis* is used in China to treat burns and is also used for the same purpose in Russia and by the Zulus.

In Japan *Aloe arborensis* is used, and also *Aloe saponaria* for gastrointestinal complaints burns, wounds, insect bites and athletes foot. The Greeks and Romans in the first century AD knew of Aloe, and it was specifically written up by Dioscoroides. Pedanius Dioscoroides was a Greek physician and pharmacologist whose dates are approximately 40AD to 90AD and whose work *De materia medica* was the foremost classical source of modern botanical terminology and the leading pharmacological text for 16 centuries. The English version of this, published in 1934, was called *The Green Herbal of Dioscoroides*. He traveled with the Roman armies and was able to study plants in many parts of the ancient world. He recommended Aloe as a purge, and to treat wounds, mouth infections, to soothe itching and to cure sores.

## Aloe Plants and Plantation

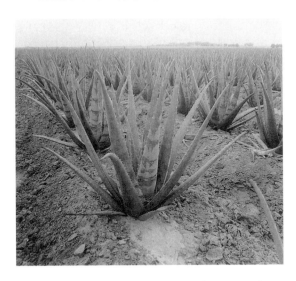

Figure 1. Photograph of the *Aloe vera* plant.

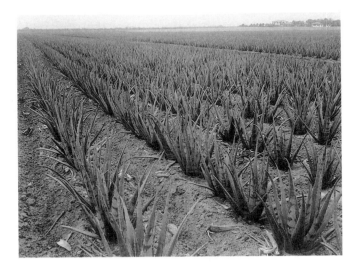

Figure 2. Photograph of the *Aloe vera* plantation.

Coming to the present millennium, the Spanish took Aloe to the New World possessions in South America and the Caribbean. Moving up to North America, Aloe came to be used in Middle America and the West Indies and it is now used widely in Western Society in home-opathy and herbalism. Medical use is especially widespread in Florida. It is grown on a substantial scale in the Rio Grande Valley of South Texas, Florida and Southern California.

One American company concerned with Aloe has listed over 100 medical disorders which have been treated with Aloe, an amazing number for just one therapeutic product.

## Evidence for Aloe's medical actions - the testimonial approach

Quite a number of these are listed below. They range from some relatively trivial conditions which might very well be treated effectively in other ways, to some extremely serious or fatal conditions. With the latter, proponents of Aloe have often been informed by some orthodox medical experts that the claims being made are out of order, insuffi-ciently substantiated, emotive or fanciful. Indeed, what is undoubtedly true about this is that both the folk-medicine accounts and also some modern articles which contain claims about the efficacy of Aloes, are based upon information which orthodoxy will always dub as being "anecdotal", meaning that they are based upon stories of successful treatment which do not bear the stamp of orthodox medical rigor, as to the conditions of the study, and it is easy, therefore for disbelieving orthodox doctors to cry unsubstantiated in relation to these accounts and therefore to write dismissively about Aloe and to thoroughly discount the claims made. Of course, if one is a patient suffering from a serious chronic disease which has no reliable "cure" in orthodox medicine and one hears of another patient with the same or similar condition getting well through taking Aloe vera, then one may well not allow oneself to be put off from the use of Aloe at all by the disbelief of some orthodox medical men. It appeals to one as a chance of getting well, as, indeed, it should. If one sees a possible chance of recovery is one actually going to forego that chance just because, perhaps, no one up to now has proved the case rigorously. There is an inherent appeal in medicine in whichever discipline one works, in adopting an approach which applies a lower standard of proof sometimes. One should not do this all the time, but on occasion, one may put oneself in a position to take a creative and/or intuitive leap in medical thought by temporarily lessening the demands for rigorous proof of everything before it is used. If you give yourself permission not to have to rigorously prove each laborious step by laborious step, then the creative leap may be more probable. No-one denies that it will require to be proved afterwards. The interests of the patient are, and remain, paramount but the Practitioner may take an action on the patient's behalf which he feels has a 95% rather than a 100% chance of benefit, or perhaps only an 80% chance, or even a 50% chance, and the patients will usually agree that they want the treatment so long as it is a treatment devoid of any potential harm. Orthodox treatment may also permit the use of treatment which has a 50% success rate, but usually, only if that success-rate has first of all been measured and proved. Because remedies which come out of folk medicine often lack the rigorous trials, their use may be accompanied by uncertainty according to the standards of biomedical science. The point is, it is better to use such medicines and accept the uncertainty than to forego their use, while, nonetheless, encouraging the setting up of full trials.

The older story of Aloe is full of these "unsubstantiated reports", as people in a very wide range of countries have experimented with Aloe as a medicine without having the backup of rigorous scientific trials. There are a great many folk medicines like that where the only evidence of effectiveness is from uncontrolled experiments and stories of efficacy passed on in folklore fashion from one generation to the next.

## Folk medicines are usually real medicines

However, folk medicines, which are passed down by generations of grandmothers all over the world, are rarely found to be ineffective as remedies when they are properly and fully investigated by modern medical science. This knowledge of medicines is not something generated by chance, nor is it the result of any body's vague whim or fancy. Rather, it is the distillation of experience down through the centuries and is certainly not to be scoffed at. True, folk medicines do not come ready-provided with the results of large double-blind studies to prove their effectiveness, but this merely proves that there are ways of knowing things other than, or in addition to, the analytical ways of modern science. There again, the swell of assertions about the efficacy of Aloes, is particularly strong and persistent. They just will not go away, and anyone who wishes to deny that efficacy faces a vast array of claims from people who have tried Aloe to heal themselves and who seem to report nothing but success. Many books contain a short account of scientific work but are made up principally of reports of enormous benefits from Aloe vera backed up only by information which falls well short of what would be required for establishing drug efficacy with scientific rigor. There is no question that the flood of assertions from users about the efficacy of Aloe is overwhelming, seems to be becoming more so, and simply will not go away.

## The symbolism of Aloe

Aloe has been associated with a certain somewhat mysterious symbolism associated with its extraordinary powers to heal. The plant has a very distinctive symbolic association with embalming, enduring life, immortality and the boundary between life and death. It has also been noted that the Aloe plant "has amazing ability to heal itself or come back from the dead", which is seen symbolically to be associated with its ability to heal humans and, virtually, therefore, to "bring them back from the dead".

## Conditions for which Aloe may be used

Some of the diseases or symptoms said to have been treated effectively with Aloe as listed here: Arthritis, gout, rheumatism, acne, dermatitis, abrasions, psoriasis boils, carbuncles, cuts, hair loss, headache, high blood pressure, indigestion, nausea, peptic ulcers, duodenal ulcers, colic, ulcerative colitis, mouth disease, puritis, burns, AIDS, cancers, diabetes, allergies, colds, Candida infection, other fungal infections, parasites, protozoan infections, viral infections, infections generally, constipation, dermatitis, dandruff, gum sores, edema, chronic fatigue syndrome, genital herpes, gingivitis, hemorrhoids, herpes simples, and zosteri inflammation, insomnia, insect bites, and bee stings, jelly-fish stings, menstrual cramps, and irregularity, radiation burns and dermatitis, rashes, oesophagitis, sprains, seborrhea, sunburn, tendentious, ulceration generally, vaginitis, varicose veins, and warts.

This list is certainly not comprehensive.

## The advent of scientific research on Aloe - the availability of biomedically acceptable proof

However, whilst the public in a great number of countries have continued and expanded their use of Aloe during the last 50-60 years, a very significant level of interest has been established amongst medical scientists, and this has led to the production of a literature of scientific papers in which the properties of Aloe have been quite minutely investigated. The results, with very few exceptions, do confirm that Aloe is, indeed, a very powerful medical substance, capable of producing a very wide range of beneficial effects. This important body of literature has not yet had anything like the impact which it should. The papers are published and are available for all to read. However, the Aloe-using public do not, for the most part, belong to the scientific research culture, making the papers effectively inaccessible to them, only limited numbers of clinicians seem to have taken an interest in the data, and the drug industry, whose job it is to produce preparations of new medical substances, will not take any interest  because Aloe is in "the public domain" and could not be secured by patents. Indeed, the impression this author has gained is that the small section of the biomedical community who have done research work on Aloe are, in effect, in something of a "water-tight compartment" in that their work has not been heeded by researchers in other fields of biomedical science. This is going to become clear in later chapters of this book, in which attention will be turned to the immune system. It is going to become clear that the ability of Aloe to stimulate the activity of the immune system has distinct implications for the larger and more general field of immunology. And yet, the connections between this work and the larger field of immunology have not been drawn.

# Two

# THE ALOE LEAF - ITS COMPONENT PARTS AND MAJOR CONSTITUENTS

## Leaf Structure

A leaf from any flowering plant has a certain basic structure, which allows it to fulfill its basic functions. Its primary purpose is to expose a large area to the suns rays so that its green, yellow and orange pigments can entrap as much light energy as possible to be used in the process of "photosynthesis" - the process by which the plant harnesses light energy for the synthesis of sugars, starch and cell constituents. By this process the plant builds up the materials of its own body and generates chemical energy for its functions. This purpose necessitates a planar structure of large area, a structure which is inherently difficult to hold up against the pull of gravity, so the leaf requires an internal network of tough fibrous material to maintain its shape as that of a distinct blade, which can be placed or angled for light collection. This network, known colloquially as veins of the leaf, or botanically as "vascular bundles" are not only for physical strength, but also act, just as the name "vein" suggests, as a pathway for the movement (translocation) of fluid within the plant. The plant, which, unlike the animal does not have blood, nonetheless does require a means of moving fluids and dissolved substances from one part of the plant to another. Because plants lose water constantly through the leaves, there is an upward current of water ("transpiration"), called the "transpiration current". Minerals also have to be transported upward to the growing leaves and the products of photosynthesis downwards to the rest of the plant. Some of this vascular bundle tissue can be seen in microscopic examination of a leaf cross-section.

The leaf also has a special layer or layers of cells at its surface, called the epidermis. These are usually packed quite tightly together. These have the function, of course, to form the plant's boundary at this point with the outside world, rather like our skin. Just as our skin is bounded on the outside by a relatively impervious layer of dead keratin material, so the outer layer of leaf cells is coated with an impervious layer of non-living material known as the "cuticle". This is made up of a fatty material containing a complex of unusual fatty acids. These are not strictly waxes, but they have something like a waxing effect, as seen in waxing the painted surface of a motor vehicle, which promotes droplets of water falling onto it to remain as a discrete drop, not to spread out and wet the surface and, perhaps, to eventually fall of or to be blown off. Such is the character of leaf surfaces that they are hard to truly wet. They are adapted, obviously to conserve water when necessary - a feature very important to a plant like Aloe which is adapted to dry climate, but also to limit gaseous exchange between the leaf and the outside. The otherwise continuous epidermis contains special pores called "stomata" which are openings to the outside which can be opened or closed to control the exchange of gases like oxygen and carbon dioxide with the atmosphere and also, if needed, limit water loss.

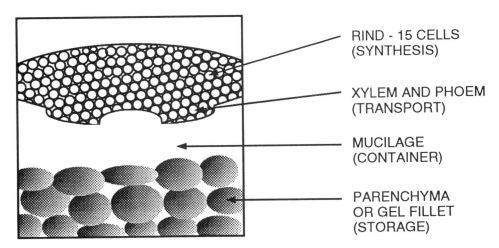

RIND - 15 CELLS
(SYNTHESIS)

XYLEM AND PHOEM
(TRANSPORT)

MUCILAGE
(CONTAINER)

PARENCHYMA
OR GEL FILLET
(STORAGE)

Figure 3. This drawing illustrates the
cross section of an Aloe leaf

The rest of the leaf is filled with cellular tissue of rather more open structure, shown in the illustration, and called parenchyma.

Immediately under the upper epidermis these cells are full of pigmented structures called "chloroplasts" are stacked in vertical columns. These are the pigments of photosynthesis and no doubt their close stacking facilitates maximum light absorption. The tissue underneath that layer, called "spongy parenchyma", has, as the name suggests, a much more open structure, often with sizable spaces in between. In Aloes, the parenchyma tissue is clearly adapted as a water storage tissue, as well as performing its other functions, and, additionally, this normally quite flimsy tissue is strengthened by some cellulose fibers between the cells.

## Localization of active principles within the leaf

The numerous constituents of Aloe which have medicinal properties are located in some areas of the leaf and some in others. This *localization* of active principles within the leaf may not be absolute. That is to say, it is possible that every part of the leaf contains at least a trace of *all* its main constituents. There is no doubt at all, however, that a marked degree of localization is a very important feature. Naturally, this tends to make it quite vitally important *which parts of the leaf* are used for making an Aloe preparation and in what proportions. This is especially true because the two principal classes of active principle that are segregated from each other in this way are very different indeed from each other and have quite unrelated types of medicinal properties. These are (1) the Exudate and (2) The Gel. Much has been written in literature about *Aloe vera* without clearly distinguishing whether it is the exudate or the Gel which is being used or referred to. Yet these two components of the leaf are, indeed, so very different, that the value of all such writings is minimized or rubbished by any failure to distinguish between them. Other preparations may contain components of both of these fractions.

## The Exudate - sometimes good if you really need it - Aloin

The exudate is a yellowish fluid which readily flows from the cut vascular bundles of the leaves. Its active principles are very large in number and comprise principally carbon compounds of the types known by chemists as "phenolics" and "quinonoids". Both of these groups fall into the really major class of organics known as

"Aromatics", a term which means that these compounds contain a particular form of ring arrangement of the carbon atoms (called the benzene ring), which form the main structure of their molecules.

## Exudate - substances with small molecules

They are substances of low molecular weight, which means that the molecules which comprise them are small and light compared to some of the other molecules which are important in the rest of the Aloe plant. Substances of low molecular weight also behave differently from larger molecules because they diffuse easily (a property by which they spread relatively easily through fluids and structures by virtue of their small size). This happens because their molecules are in a more intensely active state of movement when dissolved in water. They can also be separated from much larger molecules through their ability to pass through very small pores. This can be exploited in laboratory analysis and research in the separation technique known as "dialysis" which is used in Aloe research, and uses a membrane having pores of a known size-range. Another technique, also used in Aloe research, called the "molecular sieve" is done on columns of a support material, such as that with the brand name "Sephadex". The separation occurs as the solution of plant materials passes through the column. They become separated because the Sephadex particles will allow the molecules of the test substances to enter into their interior through pores of a known size-range. This results in different test substances passing down the column at different speeds, emerging separately at the bottom.

## What Aloin will do

These low molecular weight substances of the exudate of Aloe, belonging to the particular chemical classes which they do, have powerful properties. These are available, fortunately, almost entirely separately from the rest of the good things in Aloe, in the exudate fraction. This mixture of substances is given the name Aloin. These are often medically useful properties, but they are not the properties connected with gentle, long term healing and rejuvenation, for which *Aloe vera* is best known. Their action upon living cells may be a fairly harshly reactive one, inducing hyperactive responses, "geeing up" the system in various ways to get on and do things; but, the other side of the coin is that this potent material, when exposed to cells and tissues in high concentration, may damage their cellular mechanisms and kill them. For example, Aloe has been clearly shown to have some bactericidal and fungicidal action, and is clearly capable of actually killing micro-organisms invading, or which might invade, the human body. The antihelmitic (worm-killing or worm-loosening) reflects the ability of the Aloe material to damage the parasitic worms and put an end to their normal, biologically evolved, functions. That may be good, but it is not what *Aloe vera* is generally used for, and most people, most of the time, will naturally want to steer clear of being significantly exposed to that part of the plant. When the exudate is taken into the human intestine, it certainly produces a reaction, which is a laxative, purgative effect, which reflects its strong stimulatory power. It is not being generally used for this purpose because it is arguable that there are better, more gentle laxatives available, since the aloin fraction may produce some griping discomfort. It seems likely that the use of Aloe as a promoter of menstrual flow may also be attributable to the use of the exudate substances (aloin), acting, as they tend to do, to urge matters along, within the body, and produce a response when the body was unresponsive before. These effects from the aloin fraction are generally short term responses, just to overcome some immediate problem. Inherently, the nature of the effects of the aloin are such that no-one would want to go on using it.

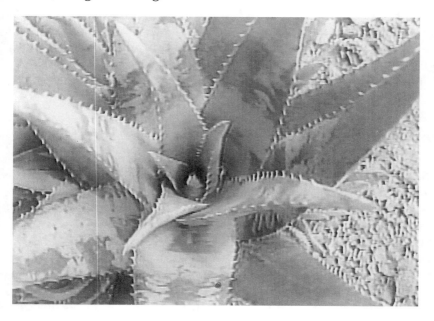

Figure 4.  Photo of Aloe Vera plant.

## The Aloin was first discovered, but do we need it now?

The use of the aloin fraction from the leaf was clearly the first useful medical action of Aloe to be discovered. No doubt, the exuded fluid from the cut surface of the leaves could easily be accessed without any special technology, so all the ancient references look as though they referred predominately to the exudate. The use of the exudate as a medicine has by no means passed away, however, and the name "Aloe" has official standing in pharmacopoeias and formularies as the "drug" derived from the dried leaf extract Today, given that most of the public who know about *Aloe vera* are not seeking the medical action associated with the exudate, most manufacturers of commercially available preparations of Aloe vera seek to exclude the aloin from the product or at least minimize it.

## The Gel

The gel is the inner parenchyma tissue of the Aloe leaf. It is the part of the leaf which, in this particular type of plant, is specialized for reserve water-holding to meet the plant's need in the dry conditions in which it grows best. The gel can be accessed by slitting the leaf through, then separating the upper and lower surfaces. The gel can then be scraped off, or rolled out of the leaf. Among home remedies, the slit leaf was strapped onto the affected part to expose the surface tissue of the patient to the gel. The presence of this gel tissue is a characteristic of Aloe Vera itself.

## The actions of the gel - strengthening, sustaining, gentle and encouraging

The gel produces no harsh reactions whatever, being devoid, or largely devoid, of the astringent-acting phenolics and quinonoids associated with the aloin fraction. Its effects and actions upon cells and tissues and of the body as a whole are gently strengthening, sustaining and encouraging towards cellular activity rather than forcing it. These words are chosen carefully by the present author and they amount to much more than just the "generalized comment" about Aloe's actions which are found in many popular books and papers about *Aloe vera*. In such writings many unsupported and generalized enthusiastic statements may be made, even though they may be quite true, without proper scientific support. In reaching the particular words strengthening, sustaining, gentle and encouraging, the author has made a distillation of the essence of the scientific literature about the actions of *Aloe vera* gel and these are his overall conclusions. In the subsequent sections of this book it will be progressively revealed that just how the above conclusion has been distilled out of the myriad actions reported for the active principles of the gels of various Aloes in scientific papers. But what it means is that the all-important active principles of Aloe, required to produce the medical effects being looked for today in Western Society are present in the gel, not the exudate. This is true whether the user employs the *Aloe vera* in a health food context, a herbalist context or a Homoeopathic context. These same active principles are also present, of course, in whole leaf extracts, because these incorporate the gel.

## Anti-Inflammatory actions

The actions of the gel of Aloes are many of them exercised through an anti-inflammatory effect. This is the calming and soothing of inflamed tissue, bringing a most gratifying reduction in pain and damage, whatever the cause of the inflammation, be it burns, wounds from physical injury, exposure to corrosive chemicals, radiation damage or an infection. There are, of course, almost endless reasons why an inflammation can occur. Many named illnesses have an inflammatory component, such as arthritis, Crohn's disease and colitis, Allergic conditions, in their reactive phases, are always inflammatory, and these include such named conditions as hay fever, and may relate to asthma, which usually has a distinct allergic component. Any chronic illness which may have steroids administered to it in orthodox medicine in an anti-inflammatory role, may be reasonably expected to respond to a potent natural anti-inflammatory used instead of the steroids. Naturally, a herbal product which has clearly substantiated anti-inflammatory effects will be reported as benefiting a very wide range of named conditions and symptoms, just through its powers to effect this one action. There are some instances in which, even in the most rigorous tests, natural anti-inflammatories can equal modern anti-inflammatory drugs in their potency of action. Where this happens a natural preparation, such as *Aloe vera*, is, of course, vastly superior overall because, unlike any chemical drug (e.g.non-steroidal anti-inflammatories), it contains nothing which is a toxin to the body and nothing which may be a problem to get rid of afterwards, while the Aloe offers many other important active principles and effects to *heal positively* and to *sustain recovery*, once the inflammation has been dealt with.

## Healing action

Another most important effect of Aloe gel is a very marked and well substantiated promotion of healing in damaged tissue. This will be demonstrated and discussed later. It can be applied most obviously to the healing of wounds and ulcers. And yet, wherever body cells and tissues have been damaged, for example, by infection, a healing process is needed afterwards. In chronic disease, internal toxins cause cell death and the degeneration of tissue areas. Recovery from chronic disease, where tissue has died, and perhaps been replaced by fibrous connective tissue, it is not always possible to effect healing in all areas, but where it is, the components of *Aloe vera* gel seem very likely, from their reported actions, to be involved in that healing process. Once again, one can see the likelihood of *Aloe vera* being reported, as it has been, as benefiting lists of diseases as long as your arm, simply because it successfully induces the replication of cells which is necessary for healing damaged areas.

## Increased phagocytosis, detoxification and cleansing actions

Also, another most important effect of Aloe is a very marked and well substantiated promotion of "phagocytosis", which is a part of the cellular process by which the immune system mops up and banishes from the body, bacteria and other infective agents and other debris, such as arises when tissue cells die. Aloe is, as we shall see in detail later, a general stimulant and regulator of immune system action, and that is a feature of Aloe's active principles which is very close to the core of Aloe's medical actions. Phagocytosis is, on the one hand, a part of that immunostimulant action. At the same time it is part of the body's detoxification and cleansing mechanisms. Bacteria and bacterial fragments and debris are clearly matter toxic to the body, which has to be removed. However, body cells which have taken up toxins and died from the toxic dose, themselves represent a hazard to the body. These dead cells get taken up by phagocytosis and the toxic matter they still contain is bio-processed and removed from the system. Improved phagocytosis is therefore one contributor to detoxification and cleansing. If one adheres, as the author does, to the basic naturopathic idea that the primary cause of chronic disease arises from the accumulation of toxins in the cells and tissues of the body, then a remedy such as Aloe, which, clearly helps at least one aspect of body detoxification and cleansing, clearly will often be reported, as Aloe is, to benefit a large number of people suffering from different chronic diseases. So, once again we see the effect whereby one simple physiological effect of Aloe at cellular level, impacts upon large numbers of disease conditions. Aloe has been reported as benefiting over 100 disease conditions and symptoms. Yet is it most improbable that even Aloe has 100 different modes of action. It seems reasonable to expect that most of Aloe's benefits will be traceable to just a few fundamental actions at cell level, which then have their effects, secondarily, on all the various labeled conditions.

## Summary

This Chapter shows that Aloe is two medicines, not one, the exudate (Aloin) and the gel. Understanding the difference between the two is fundamental, for their actions are not only very different, but also somewhat opposing. A real case that has been made for believing that in the gel there may be present traces of the aggressive purgative biochemicals that are predominant in the aloin, and that these traces, far too small to have any astringent or purgative effect, may actually contribute something important to the actions of the gel. This may be so. Some workers have claimed that the gel is completely free of aloin. Whether that is true of not probably depends upon the detection levels in the analysis. In any case, it will always be difficult to process Aloe leaves on a production scale in such a way that not even the most minor mixing of the fractions can possibly occur. So this possibility is one which needs to be born in mind when proceeding from here to later chapters.

*Three*

# THE IMPORTANCE OF POST-HARVEST CARE AND PROCESSING AND THE FACTORS WHICH DETERMINE THE VALUE OF ALOE PREPARATIONS

Post-harvest events and management are significant for almost all biological materials

All biological materials are inherently perishable, and if they are not maintained under the right conditions, or are not processed properly, then their value obviously diminishes or they may become worthless. Items like nuts and seeds and grains, in the food line, are among the most durable, being dry goods, and mainly they have to be kept out of the way of damp, insects and vermin. The value of vegetables and fruits is clearly related to post-harvest care and the speed of delivery to market. Indeed, foods should be perishable. As has long been pointed out, one should eat food that perishes, but before it has actually done so. If one eats foods upon which micro-organisms will grow readily, then it is likely to be fresh and relatively uncontaminated with chemicals.

## Growing and extracting crops for their active constituents

The same perishability factor applies to the medically active constituents of drug plants. For example, foxgloves contain the heart drug (cardiac glycoside) digitalis. Moldy rotting foxgloves would be unlikely to contain the active constituents in useful amounts. With most crops which are grown for specific active principles, the activity for which the crop is valued begins to diminish quite soon after harvest. Anyone who is in the business of producing drugs from plant species makes sure to

19

be familiar with the particular pattern of post-harvest loss which is associated with their particular crop. With vegetables and fruits it is, of course, the taste and appearance of the crop which matters most to buyer appeal, but in this field of specialist crops grown for an active principle, it is the active principle itself which matters. There will also usually be pre-harvest parameters which affect the operation profoundly also. These include the soil, the climate, the agricultural methods used, the strain or variety of the particular crop plant and the degree of maturity of the crop. Where the plant is wanted just for one particular chemical component, like digitalis, the matter comes down to economics. The buyer at the end of the line is then a drug company which will just buy the drug at the "going rate", whoever produces it and however efficiently they produce it. The product will have be come a "commodity" with no particular quality aspects applying to it and no individuality stamped upon it by the producer. Therefore the most commercially successful company in the field will be the one which most successfully optimizes the yield of active ingredient from the crop and minimizes costs.

Another specialized crop in this area is the plant *Cinchona*, from which quinine is produced. The most successful producers are those whose plantations are in the right place with regard to soil and climate, who choose the most high-yielding strains, adopt optimal agricultural practices for optimizing the content of active principle, and who extract that active principle with the highest efficiency and with the least loss. Given all the potential today of modern plant-breeding and agricultural and biochemical research, the opportunities for becoming more efficient in that type of business can be enormous. The price available to the producer for his products is fixed by the market at any particular time, and is inflexible. His profits under these conditions are therefore determined entirely by the efficiency of his production.

## Aloe - grown for its active constituents - but how to define them?

The Aloe plant is not quite in that same category because there seems to be no chance of identifying just one active principle and supplying that principle as a purified "commodity". Nonetheless, a lot of the same principles of working apply. The Aloe plant contains numerous potentially active substances. There is a difference, however, between a substance simply being present, and being able to assert that the substance definitely contributes to Aloe's medical and nutritional effects. It is obvious to any biochemist that some substances present in the Aloe plant must be there in such low concentrations that their contribution to medical and nutritional effects must be negligible. A few substances have been shown to contribute to the medical and nutritional action of the plant, and these will be discussed in detail below, even though the picture is still incomplete.

## The nature of "MPS"

In recent years, two suggestions have emerged for assessing Aloe's effectiveness. One is the measurement of its content of a group of substances called "mucopolysaccharides", abbreviated "MPS", and the second is a fraction of the soluble solids of the Aloe plant referred to as "methanol precipitable solids", also abbreviated "MPS". So far as the first category is concerned, although Aloes contain polysaccharides, which do appear quite definitely to be involved in the physiological actions of the plants, it now seems very doubtful whether Aloe contains any significant amount of the class of polysaccharides which would fall chemically, into the class called "mucopolysaccharides". The polysaccharides of Aloe appear to fall instead into different categories. The idea of using "methanol precipitable solids" may well be a better approach, since it does not name just one type of biomolecule, but refers instead to a fraction of the soluble solids which precipitate out in solid form when a solution of the soluble solids of Aloe have methanol (which is methyl alcohol) added to them. The solids which separate under these conditions contain the principal higher molecular weight fractions of the soluble Aloe solids and among them are known to be both polysaccharides, already referred to, and classes of biomolecule called "glycoproteins" and "proteoglycans". Some of the organic acids also come out of solution in this fraction. This makes the "MPS" valve at best a vague measurement and at worst an inaccurate, easily falsified and misleading measurement of the true polysaccharide content. We shall examine these closely later. For the moment, one can summarize the position reached as follows.

The total soluble solids of Aloe leaf extract, comprise:

1) Low molecular weight fraction (mainly not precipitated with methanol) and

2) Higher molecular weight fraction (mainly precipitated out of solution with methanol).

The higher molecular weight fraction, precipitated out of solution with methanol, comprises the following components.

2a) Polysaccharides, containing no protein.

2b) Substances containing both polysaccharide and protein elements ("glycoproteins" and proteoglycans).

2c) Organic acids, such as citric and malic acids, which are themselves of low molecular weight, but which adhere to the high molecular weight components.

There is no doubt that some of the very important elements of the biological activity of Aloe are associated with the higher molecular weight fraction which separates out with methanol. Therefore, the use of methanol precipitable solids as a measure of Aloe activity has some support. Therefore, in an Aloe preparation, the presence of a high content of methanol precipitable solids is certainly a favorable sign. At least one can say that a preparation which *did not contain these* could not be a fully active preparation.

Measurement of MPS cannot be taken as a satisfactory guide to Aloe's activity, because some of the other active principles in Aloe are certainly in the low molecular weight fraction. The complexity of the situation with Aloe is therefore that there are many active principles of different types. Whenever anyone speaks of measuring the biological activity of Aloe, therefore, this is meaningless unless they specify exactly which biological activity they are referring to and how they tested for it.

## Measuring biological activity directly - Anti-inflammatory property

One other approach which has been adopted as a yardstick for assessing the value of Aloe preparations is to determine the preparation's powers as an anti-inflammatory substance. The anti-inflammatory properties were discussed in the last chapter as being a very significant aspect of Aloe's properties, and one which can lead on and produce a lot of secondary, consequential benefits to the user. Quite rigorous laboratory assessment of the anti-inflammatory properties of Aloe preparation are available. Hence, this measure can be used to compare the merits of one source of Aloe with another, or can be used by a grower/manufacturer of Aloe products to assess how effective he is at extracting the active components of the Aloe plant for the benefit of the end-user. Once again, however, the limitation will be that only one form of biological activity is being examined. A preparation which was exceedingly rich with regard to the anti-inflammatory property might be very poor in respect of some other manifestation of the overall bio-activities of the Aloe plant.

This situation really cannot be improved upon at the present time. Certainly, that being the case, it does highlight the limitations of our detailed scientific knowledge. As has been said, we have an impressive amount of such knowledge, but here we are at the frontiers of it, because we just do not know how to give Aloe preparations a test, or set of tests, which would give an accurate overall indication of the value of that particular preparation in treatment. As the argument develops further, the reader will almost certainly perceive a likely eventual outcome wherein the key activities of Aloe would be the subject of four or five different tests, which would assess all the key attributes of the plant. There would be scope for one type of product to be found to be more effective in one aspect of treatment and another product better for another aspect of treatment. Moreover, with the "goal posts" defined in this way, manufacturers would be more able to set up goal-directed research and development programs aimed at optimizing all the various parameters that can be controlled in the growing, harvesting, processing and distribution of Aloe products. This author expresses the opinion that this will happen in time. The results will almost certainly be of great benefit to the end-user, since competition, in which all the most desired features of the products can be known and defined, will tend to force quality standards upwards. Producers will have to meet, under those conditions, higher and higher standards, to stay with the leaders in the field. This has already started to happen in the hands of researchers, who have developed an assay which tests wound-healing power and one which tests the level of activity of the immune cells in the skin.

We now leave the question of quality standards for the present in order to look at one of the plantation management factors and to consider the post-harvest care and processing operations as they now are, bearing in mind that the quality tests that have been outlined are currently the best that the producer has available to him.

## Crop Maturity

Firstly, it has been made very clear that the Aloe plant must be at a certain stage of maturity in order to obtain good therapeutic results, and severe disappointment has been reported from using immature plants. This could well be a significant factor in producer's economics, since leaving plantation plants in the soil for longer without harvesting them tends to cost money. Certainly, if there is any conflict between maximum quantitative yield of the plant and the quality of what is extracted, then this usually tends to become a significant question in production economics. If there is a financial temptation for the grower to hurry the harvest and produce Aloe products of lower potency, then one would expect that some producers would sometimes yield to it, given the absence of control. Only the producers concern for the long-term reputation of his products would induce him to leave the crop in the ground for longer under these circumstances, while the fly-by-nights would just be content to market products of lower potency. The literature does not reveal to what extent this question is a factor in the industry, but the importance of maturity of crop, in the overall equation, is clear. Newly planted Aloe takes from 1-1/2 to 3 years to come to maturity for harvest, depending upon the climate and growing conditions.

## Harvest and post-harvest

Given good and mature crop, the harvesting of the Aloe takes the form of cutting the leaves. It is clear that what then happens in the next few hours after cutting is crucially important. A quote from one American Company, describing their process says, "Compositional changes, while not significant in the chemical make-up of the product, resulted in great degrees of biological activity losses". This indicates that substances which are among the active principles can undergo inactivation, just as enzymes undergo inactivation, without producing much, if any, change in the analytical parameters likely to be recorded by chemists. Inactivation of an active principle would inevitably involve chemical change, but this can clearly be of such a subtle nature that an analytical chemist does not see it unless the type of change is known and his attention is drawn specifically to it. The inactivation of an enzyme does not stop the enzyme protein from analyzing as protein; maybe only the shape of the protein molecule changes (conformational change), and the inactivation of the active principles of Aloe, at least among the higher molecular weight components, may be of this same kind.

One American Company reports that according to their measures of biological activity, which center upon the anti-inflammatory property, the activity in the leaves is stable at ambient temperature for 6 hours after cutting. Activity then drops and is completely lost after 24 hours. This can be slowed down by refrigeration. They consider that the deterioration is due to enzyme action and that to some extent it is due to bacterial action. They report that the gel is rather more stable when removed from the leaves than it is when left *in situ*, within the leaves. There is marked likelihood of bacterial contamination from the leaf surface reaching the product, so the leaf surface is treated with an antibacterial chemical.

## Processing the Aloe - Producing Gel

The gel is then separated from what is called the "rind" of the leaf. This comprises the outer skin, the tough ends and the vascular structure of the leaf containing the aloin. This first step is to trim the tips and bases from the leaves, as these contain high concentrations of the aloin. The intact "filet" may be separated by manual cutting. Alternatively, when the process is mechanised the leaves are then fed into a gel extractor which first splits the leaves into two equal halves longitudinally, using a fixed stainless steel blade. The gel is then rolled from the "rind" by passing between textured stainless steel rollers.

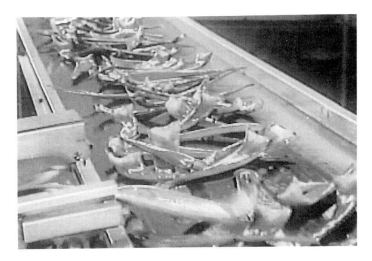

Figure 5. The photograph shows the excised gel of the leaf, or "filet", as it is called, ready for processing.

The inner parenchyma tissue of the leaf is not merely gel, but is held rigid by the fibrous cellulose cell walls. When the gel is first separated from the leaf it is very similar to a fish fillet in that it is rigid enough to be removed from the rind in one piece. The cellulose fibers are then removed from the gel and a slightly viscous liquid results. The whole process must be complete within 36 hours from cutting the leaf, and there is only this amount of time available for the processing because refrigeration is being used. Clearly, this gel process is the one that will produce a material with the lowest possible level of the aloin components directly from the leaf, i.e. without having to insert a special step for removal of the aloin.

## Processing of Aloe - The "whole leaf process"

The other important type of process is the "whole leaf process". This appears to offer real advantage in using the Aloe crop more efficiently. The parts of the leaf other than the gel itself is reported to contain good levels of those same constituents which make the gel an effective medicine. So long as one stays with just using the separated gel, the greater part of the leaf is being unused, because of its high aloin content. In the "whole leaf process" there is maximum recovery of active constituents from the whole of the crop, the active gel-type principles being recovered along with the aloin in the same extract. This is a huge advantage in terms of efficient recovery, but necessitates a stage in which to "de-aloinize" the extract and make it suitable for use, with absolutely no trace of the harsher purgative-type action from the aloin. This is best done using an active carbon treatment which adsorbs the aloin substances.

In the "whole leaf process", after the removal of the tips and bases, the whole leaf's ground in a mill to a particle size of less than 0.3cm. The ground leaf is subjected to a treatment with a preparation of the enzyme "cellulase". This is a necessary step to breakdown some of the fiber and thus to make juice separation possible. As this step may influence the biological activity, the conditions for this enzymic treatment need to be well monitored and controlled. The insoluble fibers are then removed by filtration through a screen of about 0.05cm mesh size. Most of the cells and cell debris are removed during the filtration, but the process is finished off by passing through an extremely fine filter of 0.5 micron pore-size which removes the last traces of insoluble matter. The fact that in making "whole leaf extract" much of the tissue in the densely cellular regions of the leaf are crushed and split open by cutting the tissue into such small pieces, is bound to create some compositional differences between this product and extracts that just come from the gel. The result of the processing is a clear liquid without markedly viscous properties, tinged with a yellowish color, the depth of which may vary from batch to batch of the product. Flash cooling has to be employed to bring the temperature of the extract down quickly to preserve biological activity, and it may be pasteurized at 65 degrees C, and, if a concentrated form of extract is required, the concentration is done by evaporation under vacuum.

## Different processes are bound to yield products with differences in biological activity

One would expect at least some differences of therapeutic effect between "whole leaf extract" and the gel. They obviously share in common the presence of the therapeutic gel constituents but on the other hand, it does not seem to be known what additional substances might have been added to the "whole leaf extract" through having cut up so finely, and then extracted, the tissues which compose the "rind". Then again, if it is true, as has been suggested, that the presence of some low, possibly nearly undetectable, concentrations of aloin components in the finished product is actually desirable, to enhance its properties, then differences of medical effects are likely to be found between the pure gel and "whole leaf extract". One might reasonably predict that these differences might well be, not just differences of strength, but that the different types of medical action might be exerted in different ratios by these two types of preparation. The literature does not tell us one way or the other as yet; it would, indeed, be good to see some investigations which compare and contrast the medical actions of the two types of extract quite rigorously.

## Taking care of the ethics and honesty of manufacture

At the present time good and responsible manufacturers are doing their best to maximize the activity of their preparations of Aloe vera. Apparently, there are many products on the market that are not made by responsible manufacturers. This can, no doubt, be due to failing to observe the necessary precautions in growing, harvesting and processing the products. But several writers have demonstrated that deliberate fraud is being carried out by many Aloe suppliers, the most common acts being to dilute the Aloe extract with water and/or to add to it a cheap source of sugars and polysaccharides derived from corn. This widespread adulteration of a high-value product is an alarming and despicable act, calculated to defraud people who are either really sick or who have cause to worry about their health. This shows just how important it is to buy from a supplier you know you can trust. Furthermore, if your supplier is a retailer or a middleman, how do you know that the original producer they themselves trusted to come up with the goods has really done so? Given that poor products are so dominating the market, one may well find it hard to trust the supplier. The good and responsible manufacturers are, in general, keen to see all products subject to more rigorous quality control as soon as it is feasible to do so. It is worth noting that producers also make dry powders from Aloe vera, by either freeze-drying or spray-drying. While there may be added convenience to using these light powders, rather than having to buy a heavy liquid, users should bear in mind that the drying operation is an extra process, one involving the use of heat - which the active principles may or may not fully survive.

*Four*

# THE EXUDATE -
# AND THE SUBSTANCES IT CONTAINS

In Chapter 2 reference has already been made to the exudate and the substances it contains. Its active principles are very large in number and comprise principally low molecular weight carbon compounds (i.e. small molecules), of the types known by chemists as "phenolics" and "quinonoids". The particular quinonoid compounds which are usually named as the parent substances *par excellence* of the exudate compounds are anthraquinone and anthrone. As has already been mentioned, they have a 3-ring molecular structure, and for those readers sufficiently familiar with chemical formula, the formula of anthraquinone and anthrone are given below.

**Formula 1.**

Anthraquinone                    Anthrone

Whilst anthraquinone and anthrone are well known in organic chemistry, the 3-ring quinone substances found in Aloes are *derivatives* of anthraquinone and anthrone rather than the unchanged substances.

The name "aloin", which is used in a colloquial and general sense to refer to all the grouped phenolics and quinonoids of the exudate, also has a precise chemical meaning, because specific individual biochemicals are given the name "aloin", and they are derivatives of anthraquinone. To the chemist, the term "derivative of" means that the molecular structure of the parent substance has been altered - part of the original molecule may have been replaced by a different grouping of atoms - or new and additional groupings of atoms may have simply been added onto the structure of the parent compound. In the particular compounds which bear the name "aloin", the basic anthrone structure has had two hydroxy groups (-OH) added to it and one hydroxymethyl group (-CH2OH). Moreover, it is in combination with a molecule of glucose in the form which is known as a *glycoside*. The sugar is attached to a carbon atom rather than an oxygen atom, so it is called a C-glycoside. Aloes also contain O-glycosides, which are a further range of compounds with different characteristics. Compounds with multiple fused benzene rings often do have biological activity, as in the case of the steroids. These are represented by well known hormones of the body, and drug steroids. The nature of the biological activity of fused ring substances is determined by the exact structure of the fused ring system and the outer chemical groups which it carries. Digitalis, from foxglove, strychnine, from *nux vomica*, curare, the South American Indian arrow poison and solanine, from green and sprouting potatoes, are all examples of very potent plant glycosides. Since the specific chemical, aloin, is the classic and most written about member of the Aloe anthrones, its formula if offered below for the sake of those readers able to understand chemical formula. Aloin exists in two forms, A and B.

**Formula 2.**

Aloin A

## Phenolic constituents found as exudate constituents of various species of Aloe

| Compounds | Species of Occurrence | Chemical Type |
|---|---|---|
| Aloe-emodin | *arborescens, ferox, perryi, vera* | Anthraquinone |
| Barbaloin ( = Aloin) | *rborescens, ferox, perryi, vera* | Anthrone C-glucoside |
| Homonataloin | 8 other species | Anthrone C-glucoside |
| Aloenoside | *ferox* | Anthrone C-glucoside and O-rhamnoside |
| Chysophanol | *vera* | Anthraquinone |
| Chrysophanol glucoside | *saponaria* | Anthraquinone O-glucoside |
| Anthranol | *vera* | Anthrone |
| Aloesaponol I | *saponaria* | Anthrone-type (quinonoid in ring C) |
| Aloesaponol II | *saponaria* | Anthrone-type (quinonoid in ring C) |
| Aloesaponol III | *saponaria* | Anthrone-type (quinonoid in ring C) |
| Aloesaponol IV | *saponaria* | Anthrone-type (quinonoid in ring C) |
| Aloesaponol I glucoside | *saponaria* | Anthrone-type (quinonoid in ring C) -glucoside |
| Aloesaponol II glucoside | *saponaria* | Anthrone-type (quinonoid in ring C) -glucoside |
| Aloesaponol III glucoside | *saponaria* | Anthrone-type (quinonoid in ring C) -glucoside |
| Isoeleutherol glucoside | *saponaria* | Naphthoic acid lactone-glucoside |
| Aloesapanarin I | *saponaria* | Anthraquinone |
| AloesaponarinII | *saponaria* | Anthraquinone |
| Helminthosporin | *saponaria* | Anthraquinone |
| Isoanthorin | *saponaria* | Anthraquinone |
| Aloesin | *arborescens, perryi, vera* | Chromone glucoside |
| 6″-O-p-Coumaroyl-Aloesin | *arborescens* | Chromone coumaroyl glucoside |
| 2″-O-p-Coumaroyl-Aloesin | *arborescens* | Chromone coumaroyl glucoside |
| 2″-O-p-Feruloyl-Aloesin | *arborescens* | Chromone feruloyl glucoside |
| Aloeninarborescen | *saponaria* | Quinonoid phenylpyrone |
| Asphodeli | *saponaria* | Anthraquinone-anthrone |
| Biantraquinoid Pigment B | *saponaria* | Bisanthrone |
| Biantraquinoid Pigment C | *saponaria* | Bisanthrone |
| Biantraquinoid Pigment D | *saponaria* | Bisanthrone |
| 7-hydroxyaloin | *vera* | Anthrone C-glucoside |
| 8-O-methyl-7-hydroxaloin = Isobarbaloin | *vera* | Anthrone C-glucoside |

Although the majority of readers will not be chemists, a listing of the principle aromatic compounds of the exudate of Aloe is given above. It is appreciated that for non-chemists this list will simply serve to emphasize the number and the diversity of this class of compound occurring in Aloes. Species listed under "species of occurrence" have been confined to those already mentioned in earlier chapters. Some of the compounds occur also in other species.

The anthraquinones and their close relatives, the anthrones, predominate in the above list of exudate substances. The names of the Aloe species listed indicate the species in which the substance has been definitely identified - it does not by any means indicate that it is absent from the other Aloe species. To a large extent the particular species listed reflect the fact that so much work has been done by Japanese scientists and that they generally chose to work with either *A. arborescens* or *A. saponaria*.

## Relationship to other laxative herbs

Interestingly, the Aloe anthrones are very closely related indeed to anthrones that are responsible for the laxative action of cascara (*Rhamnus purshiana*) and only slightly less closely related to some sennosides (active principles of senna - *Cassia angustifolia*). Aloe exudate is really so closely related chemically to very well established and widely used laxatives, that it need be no surprise that the best known effect of Aloe exudate is a laxative one. There are, indeed, scientific/medical studies in which the laxative effects of Aloe exudate, when used in constipation, have been compared with other well known laxatives. There probably was little need for such confirmation, but such studies have shown that Aloe exudate is up among the front runners with regard to laxative action.

## Actions of the Aloin fraction apart from laxative ones

We come now to consider what other useful effects, apart from laxative effects, may be exerted by this considerable battery of powerful compounds from the exudate of Aloes.

As stated earlier, the exudate compounds appear to be largely responsible for the reported antibacterial and anti-fungal effects of Aloe. This is fairly well in accord with their phenolic nature - after all - the simple aromatic chemical - phenol, is a powerful antiseptic ("phenolic" always refers to an aromatic substance with one or more -OH groups attached directly into the ring). In one example an ointment containing aloe anthraquinones was found to be efficacious against trichophytiasis, which is a fungal infection. The killing of invading organisms seems to be something which we can expect the exudate anthraquinones to perform.

Other reports of Aloe exudate chemicals having a wider range of effects seem to be accompanied with some uncertainty. Some papers have reported that "fractions from" or "extracts of" Cape Aloes reduced the loss of white blood cells following radiation exposure and also exhibited anti-tumor activity. Uncertainty arises here because although Capes Aloes are mainly known in the form of preparations of the exudate fraction, or have been used for purposes that are associated with the exudate fraction, it is possible that the particular preparations that were used also contained elements of the whole leaf. The whole leaf and gel fractions of some species do have radiation protection and anti-tumor activity, so it is not proven here that the exudate substances were responsible for the effects observed.

## Effect upon the stomach

However, one useful action can be ascribed with some confidence to one of the exudate compounds. Aloenin, which is not an anthrone or anthraquinone, but rather a "quinonoid phenylpyrone", and is definitely a member of the exudate group of phenolic compounds, has a definite action in inhibiting gastric secretion. Aloe gel also contains a substance or substances which inhibit gastric secretion. These findings seem to make the Aloe plant, exudate and gel, a likely effective remedy for hypersecretion of the stomach juice (i.e. hyperacidity) and through this action, is likely to alleviate problems of gastric and duodenal ulcers which can be aggravated by excess acidity. This property, combined with the known property of Aloe for the active promotion of healing in damaged tissues, seems quite enough to account for the reported help from Aloe in the healing of ulcers, especially peptic (i.e. stomach) ulcers. One recalls here that "stomachic" use was among the uses of Aloe recorded in ancient Persia.

There is room to be mildly surprised that a component of Aloe exudate actually calms down an overactive stomach, since most of the effects of the rather chemically aggressive exudate compounds are to induce an *active*, even a *hyperactive* response. The effect is associated, so far, only with the one phenolic compound, aloenin, which is chemically rather different from the markedly bio-aggressive anthraquinones.

Aloenin appears to occur principally in Aloe arboresceus rather than Aloe vera.


## Use in skin conditions - but care is needed

Another medical use of the exudate compounds has been in the treatment of psoriasis, and the use of anthraquinones for this purpose has been tried using a number of different plant sources. It is once again mildly surprising that anthraquinones do not further irritate the already highly irritated tissues of the skin in psoriasis, since, in other contexts anthraquinones have been found to cause skin rashes and to generate skin allergic responses. They have also been found to increase the production of the series 2 prostaglandin hormones which are known to be pro-inflammatory. One suggestion that has been offered to offset this is that certain components of the anthraquinone fraction can be anti-inflammatory. But this is an area of uncertainty where the evidence is not clear cut and the effects of the aloin fraction upon inflammation may very well be mixed.


## Do beneficial traces of the aloin fraction remain in gel and whole leaf extracts?

The summary of Chapter 2 considered the possibility that in the gel there may be present traces of the aggressive purgative biochemicals that are predominant in the aloin, and that these traces, far too small to have any astringent or purgative effect, may actually contribute something important to the actions of the gel. This is possible and in many ways an attractive idea. The literature of Aloe, which contains many references to difficulty in defining the real active principles, often refers to "synergistic" properties, whereby some components of the plant work together with other components, to produce effects greater than those which all the isolated components could have produced. This is the basic idea of "synergy", namely that, so far as responses and biomedical effects are concerned, the whole is in some way much greater than the sum of its parts. The literature does, indeed, contain a number of specific references to the likelihood that Aloe gel does contain some minor quantities of anthraquinones and related com-pounds, such as barbaloin and aloe-emodin, at concentrations where they are devoid of over-stimulatory, chemically aggressive properties. Indeed, during commercial processing of Aloe, it is virtually impossible to prevent some contamination of the gel with just a little of the exudate fraction. It is just that opinion differs as to whether the exudate components in the gel should be seen just as an unwanted contaminant or whether they should be welcomed in the tiny quantities in which they occur, for their positive effect in enhancing the effectiveness of the main leaf components. One author suggests that there may be a specific synergy (i.e. working together) between the trace quantities of exudate compounds and the polysaccharide fraction of the gel.

At the present moment in Aloe research, it seems quite highly probable, but by no means proven, that minor levels of exudate compounds in the gel or whole leaf extract, will contribute to biological activity. But this matter, being uncertain, cannot be defined. If there is truth in the idea, then no guidance is available to manufacturers as to how to so control the exudate type compounds entering into the gel as to maximize their beneficial effects. Which of the individual compounds should be encouraged and which excluded? The accidental contamination of the gel with exudate during processing might just happen to produce the most desirable mix, but the greater chance is that it does not. There is scope here for future Aloe research: another area in which the manufacturer could perhaps optimize his process to the benefit of the user.

Then again, when one comes to consider the whole leaf process, this is likely to involve a rather different final mix of exudate trace contaminants from the gel process. On the one hand you have accidental mixing in of minor amounts in processing the gel. On the other you have, with the whole leaf process, the initial extraction of gel and exudate components together, followed by their separation. The detailed pattern of any residual exudate components left under these conditions is, indeed, likely to be rather different from the gel process, and may have different merits. Such differences may be shown to definitely favor the use of whole leaf extracts, but more work needs to be done.

In the manufacture of the gel, one writer claimed that an important component of the healing substances passes from the rind of the leaf into the gel on standing. According this concept, leaf that was allowed to stand for a little while before being processed would produce a better product. It has to be stressed, however, that these ideas about exudate compounds in the gel or whole leaf extract have not been proven. Indeed, work on identifying and measuring any such minor components does not seem to have been undertaken and published.

This now represents the full extent of the studies here upon the exudate fraction. The subsequent chapters will concentrate on the other fractions of the leaf identifiable in the gel and whole leaf extracts. This is justified, because the things which the end user most wants Aloe to do are associated with these other fractions. At this point, one can put the exudate and its aloin into the back of one's mind as not being what the people want. But perhaps one should not quite set it aside completely, just in case those traces of it which find their way into the gel and into whole leaf extracts should prove important.

*Five*

# THE GEL AND/OR WHOLE LEAF
# EXTRACTS AND THEIR CONSTITUENTS

## Gel and Whole Leaf Extracts

This chapter is concerned with the non-exudate constituents of the leaf. Most American work has been done with gel but where work has been done on whole leaf extracts that have been treated for removal of the aloin, the rind of the leaf is considered to contribute extra quantities of much the same substances which are present in the gel. Perhaps the leaf rind which has been de-aloinized might contribute some unknown substances to an extract in addition to those that are present in the gel. This specific point does not seem to have been investigated.

In this chapter we are not concerned primarily with the biomedical actions of the gel or of the whole leaf extracts. Instead we are concerned here mostly with the chemical components of aloe gel and extracts, so that we know which substances are involved. There are many simple compounds of low molecular weight present, and it will be simplest to mention their likely biomedical effects here. The higher molecular weight fraction of the gels and extracts are probably more complex and also more significant. Therefore, this higher molecular weight fraction will be described in the present chapter and a discussion of its biomedical effects will be reserved to be fully discussed later, when the control mechanisms of the body at cellular level have been examined and when the functioning of the immune system has been considered.

## Different from many other plant juices

There is, of course, a great deal of knowledge and experience available relating to plant juices and extracts. The first thing to observe about the fluid from *Aloe vera* gel is, compared with most plant juices and extracts, it is a very thin fluid containing only a very low concentration of soluble solids. Plant juices and extracts made from forage crops, such as grass or lucerne, normally have a much higher concentration of soluble solids, perhaps in the region of 7 to 10% by weight, compared to the concentration in *Aloe vera* gel of only 0.6%. This may be fairly ascribed to the fact that the *Aloe vera* gel is a water-storage part of the plant, comprising some quite specialized water storage cells, which have to be ruptured in the course of collecting the fluid. Compared to the operations of pulping grass or lucerne, there is likely to be relatively little breakage of the normal photosynthetic cells of the green leaf, so there can be presumed to be much less release of the internal contents of the cells of the normal photosynthetic parenchyma of the leaf tissue. The pulping and expressing of plant juice, which is normally accompanied by much crushing and tearing of actively metabolizing plant cells, releases large amounts of intracellular enzyme systems, and so the protein content of the resulting juice is high. But the protein content of *Aloe vera* gel fluid is not high. Moreover, in these other juices and extracts, the release of so much internal cell sap gives rise to fairly high concentrations also of mineral salts, organic acids and sugars.

## Total solids and free sugars

According to researchers Pelley and Wang at the University of Texas Medical Branch, simple sugars are a fairly high proportion among the 0.6% of total solids in the Aloe gel fluid, i.e. 0.28% by weight, or almost half of the total dissolved substances of the fluid. These simple sugars have been analyzed as predominately glucose (about 95% of them), with 5% of fructose, which is fruit sugar. Having accounted for 100% of the simple free sugars in this way, there would appear to be little scope for finding any other simple sugars such as mannose, xylose, arabinose, rhamnose or di-trisaccharides. It is clear that any of these that are present in the free state must be there in only trace concentrations. So far as glucose and fructose are concerned, it would seem that one can virtually forget them as significant contributors to Aloe's unique biomedical actions. Glucose is such a common sugar and its properties are so well-known that it is not credible that a 0.28% solution of glucose could have significant effects. For example, an individual consuming

50ml of gel fluid per day will be consuming only 133mg of glucose and 7mg of fructose from the Aloe source. Compared with, say, the 50g of glucose that is taken for the glucose tolerance test, the amount is clearly quite negligible.

## Free form amino acids

Dismissing free sugars as a significant factor, the gel fluid contains amino acids. Different authors have reported finding them, from 17 to 20 in number, but then plant biochemists would expect almost any plant juice to contain them, for they are, of course, the precursors of plant proteins. One author reports that arginine was the most abundant of them while another that aspartic acid, glutamic acid, serine and histidine were the most abundant. The literature shows up some uncertainty among researchers as to whether any of these amino acids can have specific biomedical activities ascribed to them. One author considers that they contribute to the wound-healing property of Aloe and another that they contribute to the stimulation of phagocytosis which Aloe produces. The latter property was being ascribed to the two individual amino acids cysteine and proline. The difficulty with these ideas as an approach to explaining the actions of Aloe is that any effect of the amino acids would have to be rather non-specific, and, since virtually all plant extracts contain free amino acids, it is hard to see just how this sort a theory would even begin to explain the individuality of Aloe, and its near-uniqueness of action. Moreover, a great many of our foods contain some free amino acids, and, whether our digestive system is working well or not, some considerable quantities of free amino acids are always being generated in our intestines. True, one cannot reject the amino acid theory out of hand, because there is no doubt that individual free amino acids can have therapeutic effects when given in quantities ranging from 1g to 3g per day. Once again, given that the total solids in a 50ml dose of Aloe vera gel fluid at a 0.6% concentration would be only 300mg and that free amino acids cannot possibly represent more than a trace percentage of those solids, the amino acid theory comes to look very tenuous, indeed.

## Organic acids

The next group of substances we may consider is the organic acids, i.e., acids like lactic, citric, isocitric, malic, succinic etc. According to researchers Pelley and Wang these amount to 0.143% of the gel fluid, considerably higher than any possible concentration of free amino acids. Nonetheless a 50ml dose of Aloe gel fluid would only yield just over 70mg of this whole fraction, which is the sum total of all the organic acids present. Certainly, they are substances not noted for having any very marked physiological effects when taken by mouth. Nutritionists very frequently use mineral citrates as nutritional supplements. In this context some 3000mg/day of citrate may be given just as a carrier for the mineral being supplemented and the intake of citrate can rise in some instances to 6000mg/day. These levels of intake do not produce any known physiological effects, and, indeed, none would be expected, since the human adult produces and destroys a very large amount of citric acid each day, possibly as much as 1000g per day, a quantity which makes the above administered doses negligible. In this context, any contribution of citric acid to the body via Aloe gel fluid appears completely negligible. The same is true of the other organic acids named above, because they are all interconverted in sequence in a key metabolic cycle within the body known as the Krebs cycle, or Citric Acid Cycle.

## Special mineral salts of organic acids

Some of the substances in Aloe claimed by researchers to have phys-iological actions are mineral salts of organic acids. Some Japanese researchers led by Nishioka found a stimulant effects from *A. vera* extracts on the excised heart muscle of laboratory animals and identified the active principle as calcium isocitrate. Also, several Japanese workers have identified magnesium lactate as being one of the substances in Aloe which inhibits gastric secretion, called aloe-ulcin. These results, like some of the others that have been cited above, are really unexpected and need further explanation because of the very low concentrations of these organic salts that could be present in an Aloe gel fluid and because the compounds mentioned are by no means peculiar to the Aloe plant, being common metabolites throughout the animal and plant worlds. Because of these considerations, is seems really unlikely that either calcium isocitrate or magnesium lactate have any key or central role in creating the special pattern of physiological properties which characteristically belong to the Aloe plant.

## Minerals in Aloe Gel and Whole Leaf Extracts

Aside from the specific references given above to the salts of calcium and magnesium, the question arises as to whether it is possible that the mineral constituents of Aloe make any significant contribution to Aloe's biomedical effects. Again, the concentrations are very low and minerals are so readily available from other sources, especially vegetables, of which one is likely to consume so much more than of any Aloe preparation. The concentration of metal cations (positive ions) in Aloe gel fluid is given by Pelley and Wang as 0.103%, or just over 50mg in a 50ml dose of Aloe gel fluid. Bouchey and Gjerstad, in a paper entitled "Chemical Studies of *Aloe vera* Juice" reported upon the relative levels of the major minerals in the juice.

Using their figures, one can derive the proportions of the 50mg mineral contribution given above. These would be potassium 13.2mg, calcium 9.4mg, and sodium 3mg. These figures compare with likely dietary figures from a good whole food diet of 6000mg for potassium, 1000mg for calcium and 500-1000mg for sodium. Even if a concentrated form of Aloe gel fluid were used, the mineral contributions would remain absolutely minimal, with far cheaper items, like rhubarb and lettuce, being far more efficient at supplying them. The mineral contribution from Aloe can safely be disregarded as having any possible bearing at all upon the sources of Aloe's magic.

## Plant hormones

A further possible class of compounds to be considered are the plant hormones. In particular, two individual types of plant hormone. R.H. Davis and others, in a paper entitled "Aloe Vera, Hydrocortisone and Sterol Influence on Wound Tensile Strength and Anti-inflammation" state that "*Aloe vera* contains numerous strong growth-promoting factors" and quotes as examples "certain amino acids, gibberellin and indole-3-acetic acid". The amino acids have been discussed already, but gibberellin and indole-3-acetic acid ("auxin") are plant hormones which are known to stimulate growth in plant tissues. The idea that these plant hormones could stimulate human cells within a wound and so contribute to healing would, however, require a lot of substantiation. Davis and others claim to have extracted the plant growth hormone gibberellin from Aloes and to have demonstrated its positive effects upon the healing of wounds. Such a result requires confirmation, and clear demonstration of the purity of the gibberellin preparation. There would also be a need to demonstrate that the special effect of Aloe on wounds could be explained in terms of concentrations of gibberellin and indole-3-acetic acid in Aloe greater than those in many other plants. Otherwise, the special action of Aloe has not been explained. Looking to these plant hormones for an explanation of Aloe's actions has not yet been successful and may very well not be successful. However, it does appear that one must look for substances of a kind that might be effective in very low concentration, exerting a specific, catalytic, stimulatory effect. Hormones are this kind of substance, but in this case, their effect has not been demonstrated with certainty.

## The enzyme bradykininase

Next, Davis and co-authors also say that Aloe has an enzyme bradykininase. Bradykinin is a polypeptide substance (i.e. formed from an amino acid chain), which causes increased vascular permeability which is part of the picture in inflammation. The enzyme bradykininase, by breaking down bradykinin, reduces inflammation. Davis and co-authors state that Aloe possesses bradykininase activity and so decreases inflammation in this way. This does appear to be a really quite likely way in which some of Aloe's anti-inflammatory effect might be exerted. The enzyme, being a biocatalyst, does not have to be present in any high concentration. So long as it remains active in the gel fluid or in whole leaf extracts after processing and "sanitizing", it could well contribute a useful anti-inflammatory effect. This enzyme does not, of course, fall into the class of low molecular weight substances within Aloe, since it is a protein and hence quite a large biomolecule.

## Production of histamine

Another theory about anti-inflammatory action was that magnesium was responsible because it acted as an inhibitor of the enzyme which produces histamine - a powerful amine substance, derived from the amino acid histidine, which stimulates inflammatory processes. It seems, however, that magnesium in Aloe gel fluid or whole leaf extract, in common with the other minerals, is likely to be at such low concentrations as to have a negligible effect.

## Salicylic Acid and Salicylates

Another theory about anti-inflammatory action was that the aromatic acid salicylic acid, and its salts the salicylates, make an important contribution. Salicylic acid is closely related to aspirin, which does reduce inflammation by inhibiting the production of some hormones called "prostaglandins". Whilst this is entirely possible, it has yet to be shown whether Aloe contains salicylates in the appropriate concentrations to have such a significant effect, and whether the salicylates in Aloe are any higher than their concentrations in numerous other plants which also contain them. Cherries, currants, dates, prunes and raspberries are among the common foods which contain quite high levels of salicylates. Most users of Aloe products would be inclined to assert very strongly, surely, that the benefits they enjoy from Aloe are far more, and are different from, the mere taking of an aspirin or the eating of prunes.

## Plant sterols

In the work done by Davis and co-authors, they next looked to see whether the sterols in *Aloe vera* might be responsible for increasing wound-healing. These sterols are Lupeol, (-Sitosterol and Campesterol.) All three were shown to be anti-inflammatory when applied to surface tissues. However, whilst they were anti-inflammatory, they were actually inhibitory of wound healing in much the same way as the steroid drug hydrocortisone, and therefore cannot be responsible for the stimulatory effects of *Aloe vera* on wound-healing, which must come from other quite separate wound-healing stimulants. *Aloe vera* successfully reduces the inflammation from wounds but also accelerated their healing. This was something which could not be accomplished just by using steroids, either drug steroids or the natural plant steroids from *Aloe vera*.

## Polysaccharides - whether associated with protein or not

It will be clear from all that has gone before, that many of the substances that are present in the lower molecular weight fraction of Aloe must be irrelevant to its biomedical actions. Others of them may, indeed, be relevant. Davis and co-authors hold especially to the opinion that there is a "synergy", or co-operativeness of action, between all the different factors involved in Aloe's effects, which has been given the name of "The Conductor and Orchestra" effect, meaning that the whole is much greater than its individual parts. Some of the low molecular weight factors, together with the bradykininase enzyme protein, may well play some significant role in the overall efficacy of Aloe. However, the most clear cut results, and the most confirmed results on the efficacy of Aloe, seem to be centered around the methanol-precipitable solids and therefore the high molecular weight fraction. Some idea of the main categories of these substances from Aloe was given in chapter 3, but we now turn to look at them a little more closely.

## What are polysaccharides?

Firstly, the reader will need to understand what polysaccharides are. There is no space in this book to explain the chemical structure of sugars. The reader without chemical background is therefore asked to accept that sugars are a particular type of small molecule containing carbon, hydrogen and oxygen with, most typically, six carbon atoms in each molecule. Polysaccharides are formed by linking these sugar molecules into chains - quite long chains - forming large molecules which may or may not have branches in them. Different polysaccharides are therefore characterized according to which types of sugar molecules make up their chains. They may be molecules of the sugars glucose, mannose, fructose, galactose, most typically, but they can also contain sugar derivatives called glucuronic acid or glucosamine. They may have "acetyl groups" linked onto them or not (these are a small two-carbon grouping derived from acetic acid) and are called acetylated if these are present or non-acetylated when they are absent.

## How much polysaccharide is there in Aloe?

From the earliest reports on the chemical composition of the gel fraction, there was agreement that polysaccharides were present. Pelley and Wang at the University of Texas Medical Branch have quantified this fraction, so far as *Aloe vera* is concerned, at 0.0552% in the gel fluid, or 552mg per litre. Different workers in different countries have not always agreed upon the nature of this polysaccharide fraction. Some early reports concluded in some cases that glucuronic acid or galactose were present. However, most of the later quoted reports on the polysaccharide fraction now conclude that the main sugars present to build up the structure of the gel polysaccharide are glucose and mannose, but in various different ratios. Whole leaf extract contains these same polysaccharides but with the addition of some types derived from the sugar galactose, such as galactaus, galactomannans etc.

## Individual research results compared and contrasted

Gowda, working with *A. vera*, found 4 different fractions of polysaccharides, all containing glucose and mannose, but although the ratio of glucose to mannose overall was 1:6, individually they varied from 1.5:1 to 1 to 19. Many rather different results were obtained using other species of Aloe, notably *A. arborescens* and *A. saponaria*. The latter yielded "a glycoprotein with lectin activity". "Lectin" activity is a term which implies that the substance is active in relation to immunity and the immune system.

Japanese workers led by Shida studied effect of Aloe on phagocytosis in adult bronchial asthmatics. The extracts appear to have been stored in the dark and in the cold for the preservation of their activity. They reported that they tracked down the bio-activity to "the nondialysable material" (which means a fraction separated by the technique of dialysis - therefore the higher molecular weight fraction). They fractionated the active material by chromatography to obtain a polysaccharide fraction, which was active, and a glycoprotein fraction, which was also active.

Womble and Helderman produced a paper in which they write with enormous confidence as if "the" one and only active principle of Aloe vera had been discovered. And they conclude that a polysaccharide which they refer to as "acemannan" is an important immuno-enhancer, a name which clearly most emphasizes the mannose component in the structure of the polysaccharide concerned.

Imanishi, working with *Aloe arborescens* separated Aloctin A as a highly purified glycoprotein with known molecular weight (18,000) from the leaves of the plant. This preparation of glycoprotein was shown to have very powerful bio-medical properties. There have now been many reports of the isolation of biomedically active polysaccharide from Aloes. For example, Yagi and coworkers isolated "Aloe Mannan Polysccharide," from *Aloe arborescens* var *natalensis*. The main polysaccharide ("aloe mannan") from this species was obtained in a pure state and was proved to be a partially acetylated mannan (a polysaccharide formed from the sugar mannose), apparently free from glucose. The molecular weight of this polysaccharide "aloe mannan" was calculated to be approximately 15,000 (relatively high molecular weight) and had strong biomedical properties.

## Conclusions and summary

All these preparations of polysaccharides, glycoproteins and proteoglycans from Aloe have yielded substances with strong bio-medical powers, especially in relation to reactivity with the immune system. The general picture seems to be that mannose predominates in the structure of the most active polysaccharides and that some preparations are also obtained containing both polysaccharide and protein elements in combination, and that these glycoproteins have impressive biological activity.

This is exciting work. We still have the problem that the main groups of researchers prefer to work on different species, so that their work cannot be directly compared one with another. We still have some differing reports as to the exact nature of the polysaccharides and glycoproteins that are concerned. Nonetheless, the overall picture is that the higher molecular weight fraction of the gel or whole leaf of more than one species of Aloe *does* contain strongly bioreactive substances, the nature of which are in many ways quite compatible with the observed therapeutic effects of Aloe gel fluid or extracts themselves. Hence, it does appear that, whilst we still do not have one sole bioactive principle in Aloe, the mixed polysaccharide/glycoprotein fraction comes as near as anything we have at the moment towards meeting that concept. It seems clear that much future research will need to concentrate upon it and that much may be learned, as this work goes forward, not only about *Aloe vera*, but also about the human immune system itself. Having looked in this chapter at the various known components of the gel and of whole leaf extracts of Aloe, the next chapter will be devoted mainly to studying the more securely known biomedical effects of Aloe. This is necessary because the task that has to be addressed is the relationship between the biomedical effects of this remarkable plant, on the one hand, and its known composition on the other. The eventual aim will be to get the closest possible look at just how the Aloe plant produces its therapeutic effects. At least, to get as close as one can to that at the present state of research.

*Six*

# BIOLOGICAL ACTIVITIES OF ALOE AND THEIR INTERRELATIONSHIPS

In this chapter the main beneficial and potentially beneficial effects of Aloe on named diseases and symptoms are examined. Such effects have been included only if they have been firmly established by research reported in biomedical publications, or are very strongly indicated by such research work.

These conclusions have been drawn after collecting together some 230 references to the composition and biomedical actions of Aloe, mostly in the scientific and medical literature. All the references that are being referred to in this chapter are from reputable scientific and medical journals which will only accept papers for publication after passing them through a process of peer review. The resulting analysis picks out 18 confirmed and effective uses or actions of Aloe in a biomedical context. These are presented in summary form in the accompanying Table, indicating the likely basis of each of the actions concerned and the number of references found to either confirm or strongly indicate the conclusion of efficacy.

| No. | CONDITION | No. of Refs. | PROBABLE BASIS OF ACTION |
|-----|-----------|--------------|--------------------------|
| 1 | Anti-bacterial | 9 | Direct destruction or inhibition of bacteria (aloin) Immunostimulant effect from gel or whole leaf |
| 2 | Antifungal | 2 | Direct destruction or inhibition of fungi (aloin) Immunostimulant effect from gel or whole leaf |
| 3 | Antiviral | 5 | Direct destruction or inhibition of viruses (aloin) Immunostimulant effect from gel or whole leaf |

*Cont'd next page*

| No. | CONDITION | No. of Refs. | PROBABLE BASIS OF ACTION |
|---|---|---|---|
| 4 | Arthritis | 1 | Anti-inflammatory, Healing & Immunostimulant |
| 5 | Burns | 9 | Anti-inflammatory and Healing |
| 6 | Dentistry | 2 | Anti-inflammatory, Healing & Immunostimulant |
| 7 | Diabetes | 5 | Anti-inflammatory & Immunostimulant and perhaps effects via the digestive system. |
| 8 | Digestive System | 6 | Anti-inflammatory, Healing and perhaps effects |
| 9 | Hepatitis | 1 | Anti-inflammatory, Anti-viral & Immunostimulant |
| 10 | Immunostimulant | 12 | Immunostimulant |
| 11 | Inflammation | 17 | Anti-inflammatory |
| 12 | Otolaryngology | 1 | Anti-inflammatory and Healing |
| 13 | Pain | 1 | Anti-inflammatory |
| 14 | Radiation Burns | 14 | Anti-inflammatory and Healing |
| 15 | Skin Disease | 3 | Anti-inflammatory and Healing |
| 16 | Sports Injuries | 1 | Anti-inflammatory and Healing |
| 17 | Tumors | 10 | Immunostimulant |
| 18 | Wounds | 21 | Anti-inflammatory and Healing |
| | TOTAL | 120 | |

Comment upon each of these biomedical actions is offered below.


## 1. Anti-bacterial Effect

The anti-bacterial action of the aloin fraction has been discussed already. It is clearly due to a cytotoxic effect (i.e. a "toxic to cells" effect) from the relatively aggressive biochemicals in the aloin, and so can be described, more or less, as a direct killing of the bacteria. In this respect the action of these substances would be like any other bactericidal or disinfectant agent. One cannot be sure to what extent the bacterial cells are actually killed or just inhibited from growth and multiplication, but either way, the development of a run-away infection is avoided.

It is much less clear whether the gel fraction, or the de-aloinized whole leaf extract, has any bactericidal properties. Some clinical studies have been done which suggest a possible bactericidal effect, but the matter is by no means clear-cut. Work done with a view to finding out whether the gel exerts any *direct* effect upon bacteria has produced generally negative results. The only positive results seem to have been produced using species of Aloe other than *vera* and, indeed, species outside the scope of the small range of species discussed in this book. Even with these, the reports concerned leave some room for doubt as to whether these experiments could have involved preparations of the gel containing sufficient traces of aloin to be bactericidal for that reason. Overall, we have little reason to expect *Aloe vera* gel, or de-aloinized whole leaf extracts, to kill bacteria. With dealoinized Aloe preparations, one is looking at a plant extract devoid of toxic or aggressive substances, whose actions upon the human body are, to quote chapter 2, "strengthening, sustaining, gentle and encouraging". Its constituents simply do not appear to contain any cytotoxic substances. Moreover gel fluid and whole leaf extracts, when de-aloinized, require to have preservative added to them to prevent them from fermentative deterioration. That which has to be protected from being fermented clearly does not have strong anti-bacterial and/or anti-fungal action.

What is clear from the literature is that Aloe preparations, more or less without aloin, can nonetheless protect against various infections. For example, one study showed clearly that an extract from one of the less well-known species of Aloe would serve to protect mice against infection with the bacterium *Klebsiella pneumoniae*. There was no direct bactericidal, or antibiotic effect, however, and the action was deduced to be due to a beneficial effect of the Aloe upon the immune resistance of the animals. This is an aspect which has to be kept in mind throughout in work upon Aloe, that the beneficial effects on infections of any kind, from those preparations of Aloe which contain no aloin, appear to be due to favorably affecting the immune resistance of the host animal, rather than any direct killing action upon the invading organism. Therefore, as we seek to narrow down the biomedical effects of Aloe to a few basic ones, the anti-bacterial action of aloin-free Aloe appears to belong to the class of "immunostimulant effects", i.e. effects that depend primarily upon improvement in the functions of the patient's immune system.

## 2. Antifungal Action

There are comparatively few studies on anti-fungal effects but the overall conclusions appear to be the same as with the anti-bacterial effects.

## 3. Antiviral Action

We do not know at present whether Aloe, with or without aloin, exerts any direct destructive effect upon viruses. What the literature is showing, however, is improvements in animals and people who have virus infections, through administration of Aloe. These literature references relate to feline leukemia virus (FeLV) and to AIDS. The study on feline leukemia virus is just a single paper by Sheets and coworkers, but the reported effect upon the recovery of the cats from a normally fatal disease was dramatic. This paper must be regarded as one of the most important works on the effects of Aloe upon infections. Other reports show that carbohydrates akin to those in Aloe can stimulate cells to produce interferon, an anti-viral substance.

The work on AIDS is at a very early stage and seems to have led to some over-enthusiastic early reporting of such an emotive subject. At this stage the work has to be described as "interesting" and consistent with the rest of our knowledge about Aloe preparations which improve human and animal immune function.

## 4. Arthritis

Only a little reported work has been done on Aloe and arthritis. However, arthritis involves inflammation and damage to the affected joints. The known and established anti-inflammatory effects and healing effects of Aloe appear to be involved here in producing some of the shorter term effects; but in the longer term the immunostimulant effects of Aloe may be very important because rheumatoid arthritis is an auto-immune disease. In this type of disease, the misfunction of the immune system plays a prime role by producing an immune attack against some of the body's own tissues, directly causing tissue damage. Therefore, improvement of immune function appears to be a necessary part of any recovery from (as opposed to just amelioration of) rheumatoid arthritis.

## 5. Burns

Burns involve tissue damage and, consequently, much inflammation, leading to pain. The established anti-inflammatory effect of Aloe is therefore just what is needed to soothe the inflammatory pain from burns and the known effect of Aloe in promoting the positive re-growth of tissue needed to heal damaged areas is just what is needed to secure a recovery from burns more quickly than usual.

## 6. Dentistry

Positive reports are available on the use of Aloe in dentistry. Clearly so many problems in dentistry involve inflammation and inflammatory pain, that the anti-inflammatory effects of Aloe are clearly involved. Here again, the healing of damaged tissue is needed. In one report the use of Aloe in peridontitis is recounted, i.e. deterioration of tissue around the teeth. Such a process may involve inflammation, infection and pain, and call for healing afterwards. So the key actions of Aloe are anti-inflammatory, healing & immunostimulant actions.

## 7. Diabetes

Five papers were found reporting beneficial action of Aloe relating to diabetes. At present it is not possible to see clearly how such action is exerted. Type I diabetes, which is of early onset and which is insulin-dependent, certainly involves an autoimmune condition as one of its causes. This is an autoimmune attack upon the beta cells of the Islets of Langerhans of the pancreas, the cells which produce insulin. Hence the immunostimulant action of Aloe may be helping here, to normalize immune function. However, this autoimmune attack may be accompanied by inflammatory change, and in this context, the anti-inflammatory action may be important. One cannot be sure even that the site of Aloe's action is the Islets of Langerhans at all. If something in the Aloe were able to influence the sensitivity of body cells to insulin, then Aloe could produce a situation in which less insulin was needed. We have no evidence on this latter point. Finally, another possible route is via an effect of Aloe upon the digestive system. If Aloe's effect on the digestive system were to include an increased output of gastro-intestinal hormones like those called gastrin and cholecystokinin, these might in turn influence the output of insulin from the pancreas. Some herbs which are reported to benefit diabetes are believed to work in this way, i.e., secondarily through the digestive system, and it is just possible that Aloe does the same.

## 8. Digestive System

The beneficial effect of aloenin and perhaps aloe-ulcin, in reducing stomach acid production has already been mentioned. In addition to helping very directly with gastric and duodenal ulcers, this effect could well have a knock-on effect, influencing favorably all the other stages of digestion which come after the stomach phase. Moving down to the lower bowel, colitis is a form of inflammation and ulcerative colitis is a far advanced from of inflammation in which there has also been much tissue damage to the lining of the large intestine. Both the anti-inflammatory and healing effects of Aloe seem to be called for in this circumstance. The effects on the digestive system as a whole could be rather complex, however, and will be discussed at a deeper level later.

## 9. Hepatitis

One reference relates to this specific disease and this comprises, therefore, a further reference to a virus infection. The infection produces an inflammation and calls for immunostimulant action to help deal with it.

## 10. Immunostimulant and
## 11. Effect upon Inflammation

These two important effects of Aloe appear to be very well established indeed by many papers in the scientific literature. They are basic effects of Aloe upon the human body at cellular level, and fuller discussion of them will best be covered in Chapters 9 and 10. When we look closely at these two aspects, we shall be getting closer to understanding the primary mechanisms by which Aloe works.

## 12. Otolaryngology

Uses of Aloe in Ear, Nose and Throat conditions are likely to be quite similar in their demands to the uses in dentistry, in that the requirement is for relief of inflammatory pain and the promotion of healing.

## 13. Pain

There are various references in the Aloe literature to the relief of pain, but most studies have not focused heavily upon it. The relief of pain is not always easily distinguishable from the relief of the causes of the pain. Reduction of inflammation, one of Aloe's primary actions, will obviously result also in pain reduction. There is some suggestion in the literature that Aloe might have an actual analgesic effect as well, i.e. a direct influence upon pain reduction, and that this might even be the case the very moment when an injury is inflicted.

## 14. Radiation Burns

Here again it is obvious that the reduction of the inflammation from the burn and the healing of the damage, are the primary effects.

## 15. Skin Disease

Most skin diseases are inflammatory at the surface and involve some consequent tissue damage. Therefore, reduction of the inflammation and repair of the damage (healing) are the prime actions which Aloe seems to offer. Immune activity may be apparent at the site of the skin outbreak, but immunity problems appear not to be the primary cause.

## 16. Sports Injuries

Like any other kind of trauma or wound, sports injuries result in inflammation, which needs to be relieved, and gives rise also for a need for healing.

## 17. Tumors

That 10 papers relate to an effect of Aloe upon tumors is impressive. They are mostly *in vitro*, i.e. experiments on isolated cells growing in culture, or else experiments on laboratory animals. However, these papers offer, overall, very convincing evidence that Aloe can be effective against artificially induced cancers in animals. Hence, the likelihood that this work can be extended to human cancers needs to be looked at extremely carefully for its possible therapeutic implications. There are already strongly made anecdotal claims about Aloe curing cases of cancer.

When a human or animal body successfully deals with a cancer, it is the immune system which must undertake this task. Whilst one needs to be careful and reasonably conservative about such claims, the animal evidence is there that Aloe stimulates the immune system in a way which favors the removal of malignant tumors by the body's own defenses. This is backed up by other studies which confirm Aloe's potency as an immunostimulant. Therefore, trials of the very best available whole-leaf extracts of Aloe in human cases would surely be justified, especially as part of an overall nutritional and naturopathic approach to cancer.

## 18     Wounds

The use of Aloe in the treatment of wounds is extremely well documented, and there is, as a result, the firmest possible case in favor of Aloe here. Obviously, the reduction of inflammation, and therefore pain, is a major part of this action. So too is the benefit of accelerating the healing process within the wound.

**Other possible beneficial actions**

This completes the list of disease and symptom-related effects that can fairly safely be ascribed to Aloe on the basis of the reputable scientific and medical publications. If any particular disease condition does not appear in the above list, it does not mean that Aloe is necessarily of no benefit to it. It does mean, that so far as this author has discovered, such claims could not be substantiated. But other disease and symptom-related effects of Aloe may come to be substantiated in future years, making the above list longer than it is at the present time.

*Seven*

# The Fundamental Nature of Cells

Cells are the basic structural and functional units of all living organisms. This means that there is no life without cells and any living organism of any kind will be found, upon examination, to be made up of cells. They contain highly organized biochemical substances, which have been spatially arranged and linked together into structures. They are capable of storing information and translating this information into the synthesis (i.e., manufacture) of further quantities of these same biochemical substances which compose themselves. Because making these biochemicals requires an input of energy, they draw for this purpose upon energy sources derived from outside of the cell. Most typically, these energy sources are the breakdown products derived from the bulk nutrients, carbohydrate, fat and protein, and consist of sugars, fatty acids and amino acids. In fact these simple substances, derived from food, are "burnt" or "oxidized" away and yield up their energy in the process. The cell then uses this energy to run the cell's own economy, which includes the synthesis of the cell own substance. The cell's economy requires energy for other purposes as well, for example, for movement. It also can compensate for environmental fluctuations by altering its own internal biochemical reactions, and this also requires energy. Also, cells must reproduce themselves and, in so doing, pass on their own hereditary information, as well as their major biochemical systems. These mechanisms serve to ensure that when a cell divides into two, the two daughter cells are both exact replicas of the original cell in all respects.

This process of cell division obviously also requires energy - even just to constantly maintain the integrity of the cellular information requires some - while the synthesis of enough cellular substances to create two cells where there was only one before, clearly requires a great deal of energy. All these activities are packed into structural units which represent the ultimate in miniaturization - in most cases the cells of living organisms are of microscopic dimensions, either invisible or barely visible to the naked eye. Although the cells of different types of organism are of different sizes, and plant cells, for example, can be relatively larger, the typical range of size for the cells of multicellular animals, including human cells, is from 10 to 30 micrometers. This means that it would take from 30 to 100 of them, lined up side to side, to cover a 1 millimeter length.

Here, in a book which is mainly about Aloe, it now seems necessary to explain something more about the nature of the cells of the human body. This is because the fundamental biomedical actions of Aloe are exerted at the cellular level. The Aloe is clearly affecting and changing the chemical activities and behavior of cells. If we wish to understand how Aloe works, therefore, we have to understand these cellular actions.

## The structure of animal cells

The cell is bounded by a very thin membrane, called the "cell membrane" or "plasma membrane". Much of it is composed of what is referred to as a "lipid bilayer", which means that it is a membrane largely composed of fatty material, which is only two molecules thick. Embedded in it are protein molecules, performing specialized functions. The fatty components of the membrane comprise cholesterol, phospholipid and glycolipid and others. Obviously, the membrane forms a barrier and a line of demarcation between the inside of the cell and its environment. It follows that the membrane, and biochemical mechanisms that are associated with the membrane, have a large measure of control over what passes into the cell and what does not. This is very important to the integrity of the cell itself, because the cell does need to control its own internal milieu rather precisely, so that the conditions inside the cell support and encourage the life processes of the cell rather than the reverse. Among these mechanisms which operate at the cell surface, one, which is very important indeed, is the "sodium pump" - an enzyme system which continuously "pumps" sodium out of the cell and potassium in, using energy derived from cell respira-tion. It produces a high potassium/low sodium environment inside the cell, which is completely necessary for the ongoing life processes of the cell. That is just one very important example of the myriad of biochemical control operations which go on at the cell surface.

Whereas in a bacterial cell there are typically no other membranes or membrane processes with which to concern ourselves, the animal or human cell contains many internal membrane surfaces in addition to the plasma membrane. The internal membranes are so extensive that the plasma membrane itself comprises less than 5% of the total membrane surface of the cell. These internal membranes have the effect of dividing the cell up into compartments.

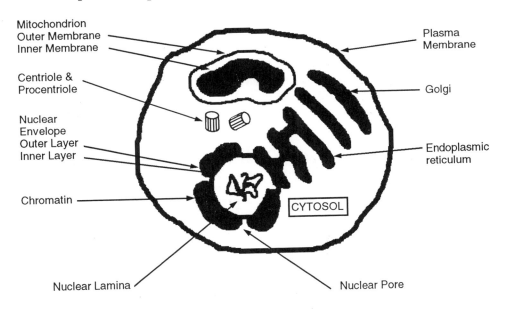

Figure 6. Diagrammatic representation of an animal or human cell showing the organelles and sub-cellular compartments.

These compartments are illustrated in the Figure above. The general area within the cell, but excluding the compartments, is filled with a fluid called the "cytosol". The Figure shows the "nucleus" of the cell, surrounded by the "nuclear envelop", which is also a membrane, which in this case has an inner and an outer layer, but leaving certain channels open, called "pores" between the nucleus and the cytosol. Within the nucleus is the all-important genetic material, called DNA, which is short for deoxyribonucleic acid. Encoded within the structure of the immense DNA molecules of every cell is all the information needed to form a human cell, and, indeed, all the information needed for the structure and functioning of each and every cell-type in the human body. This information includes exact instructions for making all the proteins, including enzyme proteins which the cell (or any human cell) makes. Moreover, since the cell proteins, in order to carry out their functions, must become located in the correct intracellular compart-ment, these proteins have to be encoded with messages about where within the cell the protein is to be transported. DNA carries the informa-tion for this also.

## Organelles' within the cell

Other closed compartments within the cell are called "organelles". Some of these are delineated by single, closed membranes, while others are enclosed in a double envelope. The closed region confined by the organelle membrane is referred to as the "lumen". The various kinds of intracellular organelle and some of their characteristics are listed in the following Table.

| Compartment or Organelle structure | Type of Membrane | Proportion of total cell volume represented | Cellular functions performed |
|---|---|---|---|
| Cytosol | Plasma membrane | 55% | Protein synthesis and general metabolism |
| Endoplasmic reticulum | Folded single membrane | 10% | Modification of proteins |
| Golgi apparatus | Stacks of single membranes | 5% | Sorting and transport of proteins |
| Lysosome | Closed single membrane | less than 1% | Protein breakdown |
| Mitochondria (more than 1000 per cell) | Double envelop | 25% | Oxidative breakdown of foodstuffs with the release of cellular energy for use |
| Nucleus | Double envelop | 5% | Storage, protection, repair and expression of genetic information, DNA |
| Peroxisome | Closed single membrane | less than 1% | Strongly oxidative reactions |

# The biochemical activities of cells

The biochemical activities of cells are obviously extremely numerous and diverse. They have to embrace the breakdown of each of the foodstuffs, protein, carbohydrate and fat. This has to cover the differing types of each. For example, among the fatty substances (lipids) it has to cover cholesterol, fatty acids, fats themselves, phospholipids and steroids. Each of these classes of substance has also to be synthesized, among them all the thousands of different enzyme proteins which the cell contains. Incoming nucleic acids (RNA and DNA) have to be broken down and the cell's own nucleic acids have to be synthesized. Some amino acids have to be modified, to make special products, like the hormone adrenaline, special chemical messengers which are active in the brain, like serotonin and acetyl choline, and the porphyrins, which go to make the red blood pigment, hemoglobin. Of course, the list is very long and the complexities of how all this actually happens is studied within the science of biochemistry.

The sum total of all these biochemical reactions is what is referred to as "metabolism". Through metabolism each cell seeks to maintain its inner composition and functions in a state referred to as a "dynamic equilibrium". That is to say, it is a state in which the various biochemical processes are continuous, the cellular structures are efficiently maintained and the concentrations of everything which makes up the internal environment of the cell do not change much. Within this state of dynamic equilibrium, the cell needs to be able to undergo sufficient change to perform its vital functions - not just its own survival functions but also those functions which constitute the role which that particular cell has to fulfill on behalf of the rest of the body, i.e. functions by which the cell makes its contributions to overall body function.

Positive functions which cells may need to perform, over and above their own survival functions, are, of course, many. Body cells become specialized quite early in the course of body development into liver cells, red blood cells, lymphocytes, macrophages, kidney tubule cells, muscle cells, nerve cells and secretory cells, and others, all of which have their own special functions to perform. These different types of body cell are in a constant state of inter-communication with each other in order to generate the complex pattern of cell activities which make up whole body functioning. Control of cellular mechanisms and activities is the key to maintaining ordered functioning within the body. Therefore biochemists have studied cell control mechanisms with particular interest, and indeed, with practical goals also in mind, since, for the pharmaceutical companies, the design or discovery of new drugs needs to be based primarily upon finding new ways to intervene in cell communication and control mechanisms.

## Cell communication and control mechanisms

Any cell control mechanism begins with some outside influence upon the cell. Cells which are packed together within a tissue exert certain controls and effects upon each other, just by surface to surface contact. Messages which are to reach the cell from rather further afield, however, must have a mediator, i.e. something to relay the message. This outside stimulus may be an being transmitted down a nerve fiber from a remote source, giving an electrical stimulus which causes the cell to do something. This electrical impulse is likely to be translated into a chemical message before the effect upon the cell can actually happen. That is to say, that the arrival of the electrical message causes the release of a special substance which then diffuses into the local area and elicits the response. Other messages which pass from one cell to another involve no electrical message passed via the nervous system. In this case one type of cell produces and releases a messenger substance which then affects cells of another type. The producer cell and the target cell may be very far apart in the body, with the messenger substance being carried in the bloodstream. This is true in the case of most of the rather well known hormones such as insulin, from the pancreas, or thyroxine, from the thyroid gland. On the other hand the producer and the target cells may be close at hand to each other in the same tissue, as is the case with more local chemical messengers, sometimes called "hormones", like the prostaglandins.

In either case, be the message one from afar or near at hand, the messenger substance usually has to interact with the surface of the target cell, and the target cell has to be ready to offer receptivity to the particular chemical message concerned, by allowing the messenger substance to attach to its cell surface. A few messengers have to be taken right inside the cell and attach themselves to a site well within the cell, perhaps in the nucleus (the steroid hormones do this), but even these have to attach to the cell surface first. Attachment to the cell surface is by far the most common method of interaction. We look next at just how this takes place.

## The cell membrane

An illustration of the cell membrane is shown in Figure 7. As already stated, it is a lipid bilayer. The illustration shows the two rows of fatty molecules, aligned to form the membrane. They become regularly arranged within the membrane because they have one water-loving (hydrophilic) end which seeks to position itself at the outside of the membrane and an entirely fatty water-hating end (hydrophobic end) which seeks to position itself at the interior of the membrane. Embedded in the bilayer are some molecules of protein. These are present for several different purposes.

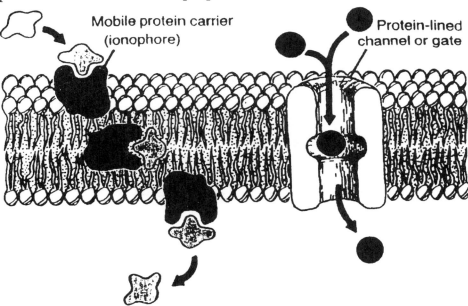

Figure 7. Diagrammatic illustration of the cell membrane showing two ways in which small molecules may pass through the membrane, either via a "protein-lined channel" or a "mobile protein carrier".

## Receptors at the cell surface

Some of these proteins which are attached into the membranes have functions which are specifically to do with interacting with substances outside the cell. In such a case, the protein will often be partly embedded within the membrane, with a part of itself directed inwards from the membrane towards the interior of the cell and another part directed outward away from the outer cell surface. The protein molecule is composed of a chain of amino acids linked in sequence, just as the polysaccharide is a chain of sugars linked in sequence. The part of the protein molecule which is outside the cell membrane can be envisaged as being like a feeler or tentacle moving about rather loosely outside of the cell yet still firmly attached to it. It is to be thought of purely at the level of molecular size, and therefore is not remotely like a grossly sized feeler or tentacle would be. Figure 8. shows such a protein embedded into the membrane. The part of the protein which is within the membrane is hydrophobic (water-hating) and it therefore tends to remain within the lipid (i.e. non-watery) environment inside the membrane. The parts of the protein which are not within the membrane, both on the outside and the inside tend to be more hydrophilic, and therefore they are in their more suitable environment outside the membrane and hence they will tend to remain so.

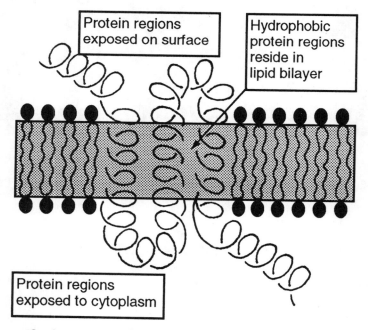

Figure 8. A transmembrane protein crosses the lipid bilayer. Hydrophobic regions reside within the membranous interior, while hydrophilic regions are exposed on either side of the membrane.

Some of these protein molecules which become positioned in this way are specially adapted to be "receptors". A receptor is a specialized protein which has an affinity for certain types of other molecules which it may "meet up with" outside the cell. So if the receptor has an affinity for insulin, it is an insulin receptor. Insulin just outside the cell, which will have come from the pancreas, will then interact with, i.e. bind with the insulin receptor, and this binding will result in a cellular response. In the case of insulin, the response may be that the cell allows more glucose to enter the cell and as a result glucose is "burnt up" faster i.e. consumed more rapidly in cellular oxidation. In the case of the hormone thyrotrophin, which is produced in the pituitary gland, the target cells are the cells of the thyroid gland and the response is to accelerate the production and secretion of thyroid hormones. In this way all the cells of the human body are under the influence of messages of many kinds which reach them from other cells within the body. Many of these cell types have developed as specialists in the production of chemical messengers which they secrete to affect other cells. Other cell types, like muscle cells, for example, are mainly "effector" cells, or cells which create an end effect or ultimate action in a series of events. The end event may be that the muscle contracts. The fact is that most cellular actions which are over and above the needs for just maintaining that cell are normally actions which are under some form of control from outside the cell itself. There are a good many different kinds of receptors known at the cell surface. There are acetyl choline receptors, calcium receptors, serotonin receptors, histamine receptors and opiate receptors, to name just a few. They are well known in pharmacology because the natural receptors which the cell produces and maintains at its surface are used as the sites of interaction for chemical drugs.

## Pharmacological action

What we are talking about here is a pharmacological effect. Substances from outside the body altogether can be introduced into it and can, to a certain extent, take the place of the internally generated chemical messengers, and can, in their place, transmit messages to the inside of the cell and create responses, in the same way that the natural messenger would do. Other substances which can be introduced from outside the body can have the opposite effect. These substances are capable of binding to the receptor on the cell surface, but instead of producing the normal response, they block the receptor so that the receptor becomes unavailable to the messenger. In these ways drugs, and pharmacologically active substances generally, whether they are synthetic chemicals or not, may either enhance or block cellular responses which are normally mediated by the body's own internal messengers.

## Where nutrition begins and ends

This subject raises a few questions about where "nutrition" begins and ends. Nutrition is normally thought of as being the supply of both bulk and micro-nutrients which the body cells need for their energy supply and maintenance of their structure and functions. But what happens when foods that we eat for nourishment turn out also to contain pharmacologically active substances? As has been observed already, fruits, such as currants, cherries, dates and prunes contain salicylates, which are closely related to aspirin. These salicylates are not required nutritionally, and so their presence in our food is advantagious. Yet sometimes the salicylates from such fruits may exert a beneficial action. Cabbage and soya beans contain phytosterols which are blockers of the actions of estrogen on cells and therefore they help to protect women against breast cancer in much the same way as the drug tamoxifen does. Is it nutrition to eat cabbages and soya beans or is it pharmacology? Plantains contain substances which protect against stomach ulcers as the drug cimetidine does, but acting via a different mechanism. Is it nutrition or is it pharmacology? It is not necessarily true that all three of these pairs of drugs and food biochemicals cited as examples operate via effects upon receptors. Tamoxifen and the phytosterols certainly do. Nonetheless, the point is that even our ordinary foods contain active principles, substances which are not nutrients, but which happen to be present and which have the power, even in low concentrations, to stimulate our body cells to behave in ways that they would not otherwise have done.

Herbal remedies are not foods. They always happen to contain a small amount of some nutrients, but herbal medicines are herbal medicines because they contain active principles. These are substances which, like those food substances cited above, affect our body cells in low concentration, having a potent action upon them which changes their behavior. This is the way it is with Aloe. There is no case for thinking that Aloe benefits us because it contains nutrients we need. It does, of course, just happen to contain some. Rather, Aloe benefits us because it contains potent substances which can stimulate our cells to behave differently from the ways they would have behaved without the Aloe.

## What is so special about Aloe and human cells?

This makes working with Aloe, and trying to understand how it works, a very exciting matter. No longer are we looking at just a mysterious folk medicine, surrounded by its history and by all sorts of excessive enthusiasms, hype, and yet at the same time, doubts. Instead of that the scientific research papers are showing us that here we have a substance which, without a shadow of any doubt, can influence the behavior of cells, cell metabolites and cellular mechanisms. As a result of doing those things it can influence biomedical processes within the body and come up with some proven beneficial influences on named diseases. Yet understanding Aloe is now quite clearly a matter of understanding the interactions between substances from this plant and the external surfaces of human body cells. Aloe will remain just a mysterious remedy to anyone who just wants to look and what it will do for this medical condition or that medical condition. Of course, that work is being done and still more should be done, because Aloe should be proved out more and more extensively in clinical trials. But when it comes to the matter of comprehension, then we have to look at just what goes on when key active substances in Aloe interact with our cell surfaces and change the behavior of our cells.

In chapter 6 it became clear that the recurring key actions of Aloe relate to 1) Inflammation 2) healing and 3) Immunostimulant effects. These are three very basically important actions. Reducing inflammation will reduce inflammatory damage. Healing processes are basic to repair of tissue damage, not only damage from trauma, but also damage that comes from long-standing degenerative disease. Finally, there is a marked effect on the immune system, confirmed now many times over. In so many of the chronic and degenerative diseases the immune system is known to under-function or to function incorrectly. The prospect of being able to influence the immune system towards regenerating itself and, at the same time, normalizing and strengthening its actions, is indeed an exciting prospect over a great area of chronic illness. These three actions go a very long way to explaining the actions which Aloe has been found to have on various pathologies. They are actions taking place at the cellular and metabolic levels and it is possible to see how they can consequently change pathological states. There are almost certainly medical conditions which are not currently being treated with Aloe (or at least not scientifically), but with which it would be possible to propose medical trials just on the basis that these same three fundamental actions of Aloe would be *expected to benefit* the conditions concerned. It will be possible to return to this matter in a later chapter.

## The profound importance of immune system effects

Meanwhile, the positive action of Aloe upon the cells of the immune system is the most positive single thing which has so far been discovered about it. Anti-inflammatory effects may ease pain, reduce damage and bring great benefit. Healing better and quicker may be a very positive thing indeed, once degenerative processes have been turned around and the causes of degeneration removed. However, the improvement of the immune system has the potential to utterly alter your health prospects for life or to save your life from degenerative processes. It is this action of Aloe upon which attention should now be focused in order to study further and then maximize Aloe's beneficial value.

*Eight*

# THE HUMAN IMMUNE SYSTEM

This is an introduction to the human immune system for those who have not previously studied it. It is offered here because so many of the benefits from the use of Aloe are connected with Aloe's special properties of immune system support, that it is necessary to give the reader some mental image of what the immune system is, what its functions are and how it carries them out.

All of us live in a hostile and dangerous environment. Each day we are faced with potentially harmful toxins, disease-causing bacteria, viruses, and even cells from our own bodies that have been transformed into cancerous invaders. Fortunately, we are protected from this staggering variety of differing biological enemies by a remarkable set of defense mechanisms. We refer to this protective "safety net" as the immune system. This system is characterized by certain structural components of the body, many of them being the so-called "lymphatic organs", and by a functional group of specialized cells and molecules which act in concert to protect us from infections and other causes of disease. The locations within the body of structures relevant to the immune system are shown in the Figure 9 shown on the following page.

## The Lymphatic System - Lymph and Lymph Vessels

The lymphatic system is a system of vessels and glands which has a function quite apart from the immune function. This is concerned, together with the circulatory system of the extra cellular fluid, in maintaining the constancy of the composition on the fluid which surrounds each body cell. This vitally important function, that of maintaining "the constancy of the internal environment", is only

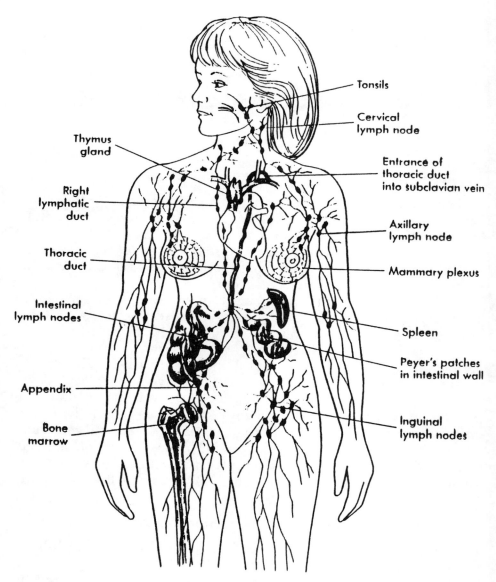

Figure 9.  Lymphatic system showing the major
lymphatic organs and vessels.

possible through numerous control mechanisms (called homeostatic
mechanisms) working effectively together in a controlled and integrated
response to changing conditions. The fluid around each body cell needs

to be moved on and changed for new and cleaner fluid, the older fluid being carried away for cleansing from the waste products of cellular metabolism. The lymphatic vessels provide a pathway for this fluid to be carried away, for not all the waste products and surplus substances can enter the blood stream by passing through the walls of the capillary blood vessels. This fluid, the lymph, which is colorless or only very slightly straw-colored, in collected into the smaller lymphatic vessels. These join up into larger vessels until eventually they all join up into two terminal lymphatic vessels called the right lymphatic duct and the thoracic duct which empty their lymph into the blood in the veins of the neck region. The blood is constantly being cleansed and detoxified by a number of organs, but especially by the major organs of elimination such as the liver and the kidneys.

This lymphatic system includes numerous glands, called lymph glands, or lymphatic glands, which are positioned along the length of some of the lymphatic vessels. A good many of them are in the arm, armpit, front of shoulder and neck regions, close to the breast, and in the inguinal regions at the top front of the legs. In these position the lymph glands are reasonably superficial. When the system is dealing with an infection, these glands may swell, due to inflammation within the glands, caused by bacterial toxins and by the intense inflammatory activity of the immune system cells in dealing with and killing the invaders. Because the glands in these positions are superficial and become obvious when they swell, most people are quite aware of their presence, having experienced some swelling themselves, at some time or another, in these areas of the body. There are many other lymph glands which occupy deeper positions, such as those located on the lymphatic vessels which drain the abdominal organs and the chest. The fact that some of the infection-fighting activities occur in these glands is obvious, and this is because the lymphatic glands are the îhomeî of many of the special types of functional cells which populate the immune system. Tissues in which these cell types are predominant are referred to as lymphatic, or lymphoid, tissues and organs which contain them predominantly are called lymphatic, or lymphoid, organs.

There are a good many other locations within the body in which accumulations of these same cell types are to be found. These include, for example, the tonsils, which are really little different from just lymphatic glands in a specialized location. This shows clearly that the tonsils are a part of the immune system and therefore part of the body's defenses. They become infected, of course, in tonsillitis, and when that problem becomes chronic or severe in the longer term, the orthodox response has been to cut them out. However, it is becoming realized that cutting out part of the body's defenses when it is under attack is not so wise, and that homeopathic, nutritional and herbal means exist by which to fortify and encourage the immune system to reject the invader without resorting to surgery. *Aloe vera* is one of those ways to fortify the immune system, and a very important one. Other predominantly lymphoid tissues are in the thymus gland and spleen. These are two discrete structural organs which have a predominantly lymphoid nature. There is also an intense concentration of lymphoid cells within the bone marrow, especially of the long bones such as the femur. Here they occur along with those other special cells which multiply to give rise to the red blood corpuscles. In this way the bone marrow acts as an ultimate or original "home" for those cells, called "stem cells" from which originate both the white cells and the red cells of the blood. The blood white cells are the same as the lymphatic and immune system cells, but those of them which are in the blood itself are, as it were, on guard and in transit. Over and above those locations which have already been mentioned, there are numerous concentrations of lymphoid tissue in the organs of the alimentary canal, especially in the intestines. Two identifiable specific areas within which the lymphoid tissues are concentrated are the appendix and the Peyer's patches. The appendix is, of course, well known for the trouble which it causes when it becomes infected, often giving rise to emergency surgery for its removal. It should, of course, not have to be removed. Often it has been long known that the person has trouble with their appendix before the emergency occurs, and timely treatment with natural remedies would overcome the problem. Of course, emergencies can occur involving the appendix without any specific warning signs, but the causes of that are always attributable to diet and lifestyle and the judicial use of herbs may well have a role in that. While no studies have been published about the prevention of appendicitis through the use of *Aloe vera*, the known mode of action of *Aloe vera* would lead one to believe that it would be most helpful in this respect, most particularly through its actions in supporting the immune system and improving conditions within the gut. The Peyer's patches are discrete and observable concentrations of lymphoid tissue within the small intestine, but microscopic examination of the walls of the intestines shows that quite dense concentrations of lymphoid tissue occur at very frequent intervals along its length and that they are virtually never altogether absent. It seems that the intestinal walls, being the body's most intimate and general contact with the outside world, having the most thorough exposure to environmental substances, have to be well protected by the immune system throughout their length.

## Special Chemicals in Immunity

There is a very extensive complex of chemical substances involved in immunity, many of them produced locally for local effects. However two substances stand out as needing to be mentioned, quite apart from the chemical activities of the immune cells themselves, namely, complement and interferon.

## Complement

Complement is a group of at least 11 proteins which comprise about 10% of the globulin fraction of the blood serum. Normally complement proteins circulate in the blood in an inactive and therefore non-functional form. Once activated, however, complement promotes inflammation and phagocytosis and can directly lyse (to lyse means to split or break, which will therefore kill) bacterial cells.

## Interferon

Interferon is a protein that protects the body against viruses and, perhaps, some forms of cancer. When viruses enter a cell they stimulate the cell to redirect its activities towards the production of further viruses. This multiplies up the infective agent so that it can continue to attack more cells. Moreover, cells that have been attacked by viruses usually cease their normal functions and are likely to eventually die, so the virus attack is very harmful to the body. Fortunately viruses and other substances can also stimulate infected cells to produce interferon. Interferon neither protects the cell that produces it nor acts directly against viruses. Instead, interferon binds to the surfaces of neighboring cells, where it stimulates them to produce anti-viral proteins. The antiviral proteins stop viral reproduction in the neighboring cells. Interferon can also cause the production of defective viruses that are incapable of infecting other cells, and it can prevent the release of viruses from infected cells. Thus interferon activates mechanisms that interfere with normal virus production and infection. Interferon may help in cancer because some cancers can be caused by viruses.

## Cells of the Immune System

Leukocytes (i.e. white blood cells) and the cells that are derived from them are the most important cellular components of the immune system. They are produced in both the bone marrow and in lymphatic tissue and are released into the blood and are then transported about the body. To be effective, leukocytes must move into the tissues where they are needed. Certain special substances which are parts of microbes, or chemicals that are released by tissue cells, act as chemical signals to attract leukocytes. These are termed "chemotactic factors" and these include histamine, complement, kinins and leukotrienes. The terms "chemotactic or chemotaxis" are reserved for chemical messengers which promote cell movement. They diffuse outward from the area in which they are being released. The leukocytes can detect small differences in the concentration of these substances and they are programmed to move towards higher concentrations of them, moving through the blood or tissue fluid, squeezing in between cells or, even on occasion, passing through cells. Each type of leukocyte has its specific functions in connection with immunity.

## Neutrophils

These are fairly small cells produced in the bone marrow at the rate of well over 100 billion per day. They are usually the first immune system cells to enter a site of infection and they act by phagocytosis. They migrate to the gastro-intestinal tract in great numbers, where they provide phagocytic protection against bacteria and other undesirables entering from the food. As part of this process, they release digestive enzymes from their lysosomes (one type of intracellular organelle) and these same enzymes can also cause inflammatory tissue damage locally.

## Macrophages

These develop from another type of white cell called the monocyte. They are large phagocytic cells and can ingest more and larger particles than can the neutrophils. They arrive at infected sites later than the neutrophils and are responsible for a lot of cleaning up activities, including the clearing up of neutrophils that have died as a result of having ingested foreign particles. They produce a number of active chemicals, including prostaglandins, complement and interferon, which play an important part in the immune process. They provide protection to the skin and its underlying layers, where they are known as Langerhans cells, and they protect the mucous and serous membranes, the uterus, the blood and lymph vessels and the bladder. Macrophages also filter out microbes within the spaces inside the lymph glands, in the liver, where they are called Kupffer cells, central nervous system, where they are called microglia, and in spleen and bone marrow.

## Basophils, and Mast Cells

These originate in the bone marrow, the basophils being motile (i.e. actively moving) in the blood and tissues and the mast cells being stationary in tissues such as gastrointestinal tract, urinary tract, lungs and skin. They can both be activated by complement or by antibodies and can release active chemicals such as leukotrienes and histamine.

## Eosinophils

These also originate in bone marrow and then they quickly enter tissues. They produce enzymes which break down the chemicals released by Basophils, and Mast Cells. Hence, the inflammatory process has a built-in control mechanism that can wind it down when appropriate. These cells tend to multiply and become numerous when there are allergies or parasitic infections.

## Lymphocytes

Lymphocytes, like all blood cells, are derived from the bone marrow. Some of the stem cells in the bone marrow give rise to pre-lymphocytes called pre-T-cells. These migrate to the thymus gland. They multiply there and are processed into finished T-cells. T-cells are one of the principal types of lymphocyte and they are divisible into a number of subclasses. The T-cells are responsible for an important category of immune function called cell-mediated immunity.

Some other stem cells in the bone marrow give rise to B-cells. These produce special proteins called antibodies, which circulate in the blood and which can combine with foreign particles and substances, neutralizing them so far as toxicity is concerned, or simply making them more "palatable" for ingestion by phagocytes. This class of immunity is called "humoral" or "antibody-mediated immunity".

T-cells of any class have a long life and are very motile, so increasing the chances that they will encounter the foreign organisms or substances which the body needs to eliminate. Their motility also enables them to travel readily to sites of inflammation. It appears that small groups of identical lymphocytes form during the development of the embryo. These are called clones. Each clone can respond only to one particular type of foreign particle or substance. Consequently, there has to be a very large number of clones to give the body the ability to respond to all possible foreign materials.

The different classes of T-lymphocytes have very specific functions. There are cytotoxic (killer) T-cells and delayed hypersensitivity T-cells which are responsible, together, for actually carrying out the cell-mediated immune response. However, there are also regulatory T-cells, i.e. cells which control the intensity of the cell-mediated immune response. These either intensify it or slow it down and the cell types are known as "helper T-cells or suppresser T-cells".

## Activation of Lymphocytes

The foreign substance which triggers an immune response is referred to as an "antigen". In order to produce a specific immune response, the lymphocytes must recognize the particular antigen. However, lymphocytes do not recognize and respond to the complete antigen, only to certain regions of its molecular structure. In this way one antigen substance may comprise several different specific regions which can activate lymphocytes. These areas of recognition that occur within the molecular structure of antigens are called "antigenic determinants". All the members of one clone of lymphocytes have the ability to recognize just one of these antigenic determinants through a particular type of molecule on its own surface. When recognition occurs it takes the form of a bonding between the specific molecules on the lymphocyte surface and the "antigenic determinant" area of the antigen molecule. This binding process depends upon the shape, size and electrical charge on the molecules concerned, and where there is recognition the recognizing molecule on the lymphocyte surface fits the antigenic determinant region of the antigen like a "lock and key", and that analogy is frequently used to describe it. The T-lymphocyte surface molecule is called the T-cell receptor and its detailed structure has been well investigated and is now well known to biochemists and immunologists. The T-cell receptor has polypeptide chains extending through the cell membrane and protruding onto the surface in the same way as the unspecified receptor illustrated in chapter 7.

Most lymphocyte activation involves helper T-cells, but before this can happen the antigen has to be processed by any of the so-called "antigen-presenting cells". These are B-cells, macrophages and other cells which are closely akin to the macrophages. These cell types break down the antigen and so process it that they thereafter present fragments of the antigen, the parts that need to be recognized, on their own cell surface. They then present the part-antigen ("antigenic determinant") to helper T-cells. The macrophages also stimulate the helper T-cells to divide. Some very important chemicals called interleukin-1 and 2 are involved in this process. This results in the multiplication of helper

T-cells. These, in turn, activate B-cells and the two classes of T-cell which carry out the cell-mediated immune response. By contrast with this, the suppresser T-cells reduce the active immune response, and so they constitute a means by which the body can modulate and regulate the immune process so that it does not rage ahead out of control.

Obviously, therefore, anything which tends to accelerate or activate the work of the T-helper cells is going to intensify the immune process. The action of substances in *Aloe vera* does activate and intensify the immune response, and this constitutes one of the fundamental scientifically established actions of Aloe upon the body. The way in which it does that, insofar as it is known at the moment, is the subject of the next chapter, in which it will be shown that quite definite stimulatory effects upon immune system cells have been demonstrated by a number of researchers.

## The Basis of Auto-immunity

In providing the immense number of clones of leukocytes necessary to enable the immune system to respond to any possible invasive antigen, the body has, incidentally, provided itself with clones of cells that have the ability to respond to self-antigens. By "self-antigens" is meant antigens which are an integral part of the body itself. This is a potentially dangerous strategy. The mere ability to recognize self-antigens means that there is also the ability to react to antigens which are a part of oneself. That truly is a horror scenario because an effective immune attack on parts of one's own body will inevitably mean the inflicting of very severe damage upon those parts and possibly, in the fullness of time, the ultimate destruction of those parts. The problem of auto-immunity, in which this type of attack occurs, has been discussed in chapter 6, with particular reference to the pancreas and Type I diabetes. However, the problem of auto-immunity is also present in the following other conditions. Pernicious anemia, Hashimoto's thyroiditis (i.e. one type of thyroid insufficiency), Grave's disease (i.e. Thyrotoxicosis), Rheumatoid arthritis, Systemic Lupus and Lupus erythematosus, sing through the walls of the capillary blood vessels. This fluid, the lymph, which is colorless or only very slightly straw-colored, is collected into the smaller lymphatic vessels. These join up into larger vessels until eventually they all join up into two terminal lymphatic vessels called the right lymphatic duct and the thoracic duct, which empty their lymph into the blood in the veins of the neck region. The blood is constantly being cleansed and detoxified by a number of organs, but especially by the major organs of elimination such as the liver and the kidneys.

*Nine*

# ALOE'S INTERACTIONS WITH THE IMMUNE SYSTEM - RESEARCH WHICH SHOWS THAT ALOE INFLUENCES SYSTEM IMMUNE CELLS

The previous chapter shows the principal factors which are involved in determining the efficacy and efficiency of the immune system in dealing with the various bacteria, viruses, toxins, waste products and debris which may enter and accumulate within the human body. It clearly depends upon the functional activity of all the various classes of cells within the immune system, including those which are responsible for both cell-mediated immunity and humoral immunity, or antibodies.

Among these various cell types and their different functions, the process of phagocytosis plays an important part of the overall processes of immunity. The actual phagocytosis step is really a cleaning up operation after some of the earlier immune processes have taken place. In the earlier stages, antibody proteins are likely to have been produced against the offending item, which coat it and make it more "palatable" to phagocytosis. Also, if the offending item is a bacterial cell, or even a moribund body cell, it may have been killed by the action of "killer" lymphocytes. Nonetheless, phagocytosis is an extremely important step and can be seen as a cleansing process. The phagocytosed item is "neutralized" and ends up being destroyed and eliminated. The digestive and oxidizing processes that take place within the phagocyte destroys the structure of the offending item and make it unrecognizable as what it was. The effect is therefore both protective and cleansing. The phagocyte may even migrate to a place from which it will be eliminated, as when it migrates to an area of pus, such as a boil, and the pus is eventually shed from the surface.

Obviously, anything which can make the process of phagocytosis more effective and more active is going to be significant for the processes of immunity. Such a substance will be an immune system stimulant. Aloe vera is such a substance.

## Scientific References to Stimulation of Phagocytosis and other Immune Functions

The effect of Aloe in stimulating and supporting phagocytosis is so important in relation to Aloe's overall action that mention is made here of specific workers and specific published papers which together serve to clearly demonstrate that the effect is real and considerable.

In 1977, Stepanova, O.S., Prudnik N.Z. *et al.* wrote *Chemical Composition and Biological Activity of Dry Aloe Leaves*, in which they reported that dried extracts of *A. arborescens* leaves increased phagocytic activity in guinea pig leukocytes *in vivo*.

Later, work was reported by Professor A. Yagi and others, of Japan, in 1985 and 1987. Writing in an internationally recognized journal dealing with the medical effects of plants and plant substances, and also in a Japanese journal specializing in allergies, Professor Yagi reported upon phagocytosis occurring in adult patients suffering from bronchial asthma. He isolated a polysaccharide and also a glycoprotein and demonstrated that they would (either of them) stimulate phagocytosis in neutrophils which had been taken from the blood of the asthmatic patients. The effect was shown to be dose-dependent, i.e. the larger the dose of the Aloe substances used, the larger was the increase in the phagocyte response.

A further reference, by 't Hart and colleagues in the Netherlands, in 1989 relates to the stimulation of immune activity in mice by local activation of a substance known as "complement" and by increase in antibody production. In its conclusions it makes reference to the "activation of human polymorphonuclear leukocytes (neutrophils)". Once again it is clear that major immuno-stimulatory activity is being reported. The same reference reports upon the stimulation of specific antibody production, which comes, of course, from the activity of the B lymphocytes, and also reports T lymphocyte activation occurring in the living animal. Not only is the reported immuno-stimulation a major effect, but it can therefore be seen to cover simultaneously several aspects of immune system function.

A further reference from the same authors in 1990, reiterates some of the work of the previous year, and then notes additionally that low molecular weight constituents from Aloe vera gel (i.e. the non-dialyzable, non-polysaccharide, non-glycoprotein fraction), contains substances which can inhibit the release from the neutrophils of those powerful chemicals which both neutrophils and macrophages produce to kill ingested bacteria. Some of these substances are referred to as "reactive oxygen species". This refers to the fact that oxygen in an activated form has powerful cell-killing activity. The irreactive oxygen species can be either the negatively charged oxygen molecule, $O_2$ or hydrogen peroxide, $H_2O_2$. These are aggressive chemical reagents, and within the body their use and distribution have to be carefully controlled so that they can be used to kill invading bacteria or cancer cells without risking damage to the rest of the body, or any of the body's healthy and functional cells. The finding that *Aloe vera* constituents diminish the extent to which these "reactive oxygen species" leak out from the neutrophil into the cell's environment is favorable. Clearly such reactive species are best confined within the boundaries of the cells in which they work. The above authors consider that the benefit from the use of Aloe in this instance is precisely from encouraging such retention within the cell. Once outside the cell the "reactive oxygen species" are free to react with any substances or structures with which they come into contact. There is little doubt that when this happens various degrees of damage is done to neighboring cells and tissue structures. This type of cellular and tissue damage is well known to pathologists. While inflammation is a natural reaction of the body's defenses, and normally should not be suppressed, if inflammation is long-continued, damage to the neighboring and surrounding structures ensues. For example, the chronic inflammation in arthritic joints, because it is so long continued, takes the form of damage to the tissue structures of the joints themselves. This is inflammatory damage. Without a doubt, then, the inflammation, which was originally desirable because it was the means by which the body sought to relieve itself of a source of toxic deposit located within the joints, has become counter-productive, resulting in damage, often of serious extent, to the actual structure of the joints. It seems most likely that this sort of long-term inflammatory damage is, indeed, due to oxidative damage brought about by the "escape" of the noxious oxidative agents ("reactive oxygen species") created to deal with the problem. Therefore, the action of the low molecular weight fraction from Aloe is being, with reference to chapter 2, wholly "strengthening, sustaining, gentle and encouraging" in its action here. The lethal killing properties of the immune cells is in no way reduced by action of the Aloe. In fact the Aloe merely encourages the retention of the lethal reagents inside the immune cell, which is the place where they can be effective. In this way the immune cell is being made more efficient in its work and the surrounding tissue matrix and tissue cells are being spared from inflammatory damage.

The following additional recent reference relates to work with chickens in which the complex carbohydrate from *Aloe vera* was found to increase the output of nitric oxide by macrophages. Nitric oxide is one of the lethal chemicals produced by the immune system and macrophages use it for killing and neutralizing harmful bacteria and for the destruction of foreign substances and debris in the same way as hydrogen peroxide is used for a similar purpose. Obviously, then an increased output of nitric oxide provides a means by which macrophage cells can increase the effectiveness of their phagocytic activity.

In addition, the following American article entitled "Immune enhancing effects of Aloe", by J.C. Pittman in 1992, is a short review and summary rather than original research. It cites that "Acemannan has direct effects on the immune system, activating and stimulating macrophages, monocytes, antibodies and T-cells." Acemannan is a trade name which has been applied to the mannose-rich polysaccharide fraction from Aloe. T-cells are one of the major classes of lymphocytes. Pittman also says that "It (acemannan) has been shown in laboratory studies to act as a bridge between foreign proteins (such as virus particles) and macrophages, facilitating phagocytosis."

A paper by Solar and others in 1979 found that an Aloe preparation markedly increased the resistance of mice to the pathogenic bacterium *Klebsiella pneumoniae*. Apparently it did so, not through any effect of directly killing the bacterium (i.e. no antibiotic effect) but rather through positive effects on the performance of the animals' immune system. Other workers have also found Aloe to have most dramatic effects in protecting against infections. One of the most remarkable of these was an American paper by M.A. Sheets and colleagues entitled "Studies on the effect of acemannan on retrovirus infections: clinical stabilization of feline virus-infected cats." In this work it was shown that cats, which would normally only rarely recover from the feline leukemia virus, showed a high rate of recovery when treated with the "acemannan". Once again, it was most unlikely that the Aloe was acting *in vivo* directly as a virus-inactivating agent, and it appeared that the effect was being wholly mediated through the immune systems of the animals.

A paper by Womble & Helderman (1988) studied the effects of "acemannan" upon human white blood cells and concluded that acemannan is an important immuno-enhancer. They discussed this in relation to specific cell types. In particular, they concluded that another cell type not yet discussed, namely the monocyte, is involved in immune system stimulation by Aloe and that a key effect of Aloe is to enhance monocyte - T cell co-operation. These authors were keen to find out whether the useful immuno-enhancing effects of Aloe occur at concentrations of Aloe constituents that are likely to be achieved in clinical practice. They wrote, "The actual concentrations achievable in man also have been shown to be in this range, further supporting the potential relevance for clinical practice of these studies". They go on "... the active substance derived from the *Aloe vera* plant, which from time immemorial has been felt to be clinically beneficial, has been shown to be an immuno-enhancing agent *in vitro* with respect to ... mixed lymphocyte culture". They end up "This drug holds important promise as a clinically useful anti-viral agent".

These scientific papers that have been mentioned here are by no means the limit of what has been written in the scientific literature, demonstrating that the immune system is, indeed, activated and supported by Aloe in a most impressive way.

## How the Immune Cells are Stimulated

The way in which the mannose-rich polysaccharides of Aloe influence the immune system cells is clearly via the specialized cell-surface receptors described in Chapter 8. These are like sensitized radio antennae, characterized by their protein chains which protrude beyond the outer surface of the cell membrane, ready to interact and unite with any specific substance which matches the way in which the particular receptor is programmed by it own specific amino acid sequence. The immune cells certainly have many different cell-surface receptors each with its own limited spectrum of sensitivity. The receptors which interact with the mannose-rich polysaccharides are apparently specific for their mannose component. Several investigators who have studied the immuno-stimulant properties of Aloe have commented upon the types of receptor involved on the surfaces of the macrophages or neutrophils. A paper by Winters (1993), after presenting experimental results, declares "These results suggest that these Aloe lectins were active at alpha D-glucose and mannose sites and not at N-acetyl glucosamine sites". The white blood cells being used in this work appear to have been predominantly lymphocytes.

The precise way in which this glucomannan/receptor interaction occurs has not been elucidated. The best mental image we have of Aloe glucomannan interacting with cellular receptors is that provided by Dr.

Robert H. Davis of Pennsylvania. He produced this in the course describing the interaction of the glucomannan with the receptors of fibroblasts. These cells are not part of the immune system, but are deeply involved in the healing of wounds. Nonetheless, the image created by Dr Davis is important, and is based upon much evidence plus some informed interpretation. The glucose part of the molecule is seen as binding the polysaccharide to protein, and is attached to the polysaccharide chain which is made up mostly of mannose sugar molecules linked together. The last (i.e."terminal") mannose sugar molecule is phosphorylated (i.e. combined with phosphate) and this terminal phosphorylated sugar unit binds to the cell-surface receptors. This is fully compatible with the observation that mannose phosphate, by itself, exerts some degree of stimulatory effect upon the cells. An illustration is presented below to show the polysaccharide/cell receptor interaction.

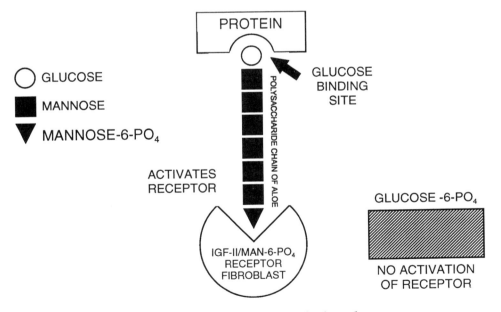

Figure 10. The mechanism of action of Aloe glucomannan, along with protein, upon fibroblast cell surface receptors.

## Summing up Aloe's Immuno Effects

The evidence above fully justifies the general statement which this author has made elsewhere about the nature of the interaction between the glucomannan of Aloe and the immune system cells. This was;

"Specialized molecules in *Aloe vera* whole leaf extract interact with some special "receptor" substances that are embedded into the outer membrane of our immune system cells. The result is that the immune system cells are galvanized into action. In particular, the class of cells known as "phagocytes" increase the activities by which they attack and then engulf bacteria, waste products and debris. This increase in scavenging activities cleanses and protects the body, with knock-on benefits for a whole cascade of different medical conditions. The literature indicates a common mechanism in this respect probably exists in both humans and animals and that both can benefit enormously from use of *Aloe vera.*"

## Interrelationships between Immune System and Bowel

To follow on from this point to study the effects upon the whole organism of the beneficial effects of Aloe is mainly the task of another Chapter. However, it is worth while to consider once more the article by J.C. Pittman (1992). He says "The most striking commonality found in individuals suffering with immuno-depressive conditions (Epstein-Barr virus, Chronic Fatigue Syndrome, systemic candidiasis, HIV infection and others) is their high incidence of digestive dysfunction and maldigestion. This has several effects that contribute to stress on the immune system and therefore its weakening."

This reference to digestive function is, indeed, interesting. One of the most frequently repeated assertions coming from alternative and complementary medical practitioners, as well as from the general public, is that they find Aloe enormously helpful so far as digestive problems are concerned, and yet there has been only minimal attention to that aspect of Aloe in scientific and medical literature. Digestive dysfunctions are, indeed, inclined to occur in the same people who have known immunodeficiency, but it really is not clear whether the digestive problems cause the immune problems or the other way around. This author agrees with Pittman that gastro-intestinal dysfunction, once established, will lead to a considerable worsening of the health status of the immune system. This happens because the immune cells are starved of the correct nutrients and because the presence of incompletely digested foods in the intestine places a considerable extra work-load upon the immune system. However, these two processes of deterioration will fuel one another. In other words, immune system dysfunction is very likely to lead to poor digestion. The digestive system, as has been explained in chapter 8, is equipped with a high content of immune tissue, presumably for the purpose of dealing with microbial invaders and other noxious and toxic items coming from the intestinal contents. Immune dysfunction could, therefore, come before digestive dysfunction, or the two systems might well deteriorate conjointly, due to their mutual interdependence.

What this seems to mean is that the whole big area of bowel disease may arise in part, at least, from immune system dysfunction and hence that bowel disease may well have to be included in the cascade of consequences which flows from having an under functioning and compromised immune system.

Please see page 123 for a list of scientific literature on the immunostimulant action of aloe.

*Ten*

# RESEARCH WHICH HAS ESTABLISHED ALOE AS A POWERFUL MEDICINE

This chapter fills out the information about Aloe's effects upon named diseases and symptoms. It concentrates upon establishing how real and certain these effects are. Once again, although this is not a scientific treatise, the opportunity is taken to mention specific papers and authors as examples of good scientific inquiry being applied to Aloe in the quest to elucidate its biomedical effects.

In this Chapter, the inquiry into the immune system effects is taken as being complete for the time being, though chapter 12 will deal with the knock-on consequences of immune system stimulation. We also omit the antibacterial, anti-viral and anti-fungal effects from this chapter, important though they are, because they too flow from the beneficial immune system effects that have been described already. Also, the anti-inflammatory and healing effects, being among the fundamental actions of Aloe at cellular and tissue level, are to be examined in chapter 11. Here we deal with named medical conditions more closely than we did in Chapter 6, and the scientific and medical work which has been done to establish whether or not treatment with Aloe produces either improvement or cure.

The medical conditions to be examined are; wounds, thermal burns, radiation burns, diabetes, leg ulcers and dermatoses, peptic ulcer, arthritis, intestinal and digestive disorders, tumors.

## Wounds

A very early paper on this subject is that of Barnes (1947) entitled "The healing action of extracts of *Aloe vera* on abrasions of the human skin". Since then many investigators have addressed the subject, for example, Goff & Levenstein (1964) "Measuring the effects of topical preparations upon the healing of skin wounds" and Rubel (1983) "Possible mechanisms of the healing actions of *Aloe vera* gel". From 1987 onwards, Professor Davis and co-workers, of the Pennsylvania College of Podiatric Medicine, Philadelphia, U.S.A. have worked extensively in this area and produced a number of research papers on the subject, for example, in 1988, "Aloe Vera: "A Natural Approach for Treating Wounds, Oedema and Pain in Diabetes", and in 1989 "Wound Healing. Oral and Topical Activity of *Aloe vera*", in 1993, "Principles of Wound Healing and Growth Factor Considerations", in 1994, "Aloe Vera, Hydro-cortisone. and Sterol Influence on Wound Tensile Strength and Anti-inflammation." and "Anti-inflammatory and Wound Healing Activity of a Growth Substance in Aloe vera". Prof. Davis's group have been very concerned with the quest to find the mechanisms of action of *Aloe vera* in producing both the anti-inflammatory and healing effects, and this has produced some most interesting findings and theories. However, the key point here at the moment is that all these papers, by Prof. Davis's group and many others, have fully confirmed the activity of *Aloe vera* in accelerating the healing of wounds and have done so many times over. The detailed work done to elucidate the mechanisms by which this occurs, involves frequent repetition of the basic experimental observations and clearly shows that the phenomenon of wound healing by *Aloe vera* is entirely reproducible and reliable. Moreover, the work done shows that the effect of *Aloe vera* on wound healing is very marked, so that up to 50% or more healing may occur with the use of Aloe than without. Therefore, this is no minor effect and Aloe is very worth while using for this purpose.

It is worth noting that this wound healing effect, which has been so extensively studied and which by now has been at least partly understood by investigators, represents a phenomenon which can be observed, not just in the healing of wounds, but also in more general healing. Lesions which need to be healed do not occur only through physical trauma, but also through chronic and degenerative illness. This fact is observable in clinical practice whenever a chronic condition which has been long standing is being treated and reversed. It is an observation which, perhaps, does not fit too easily with the concepts of very orthodox medicine, but in clinical practice within naturopathic medicine or herbal medicine, or in the author's own particular field of nutritional medicine, the reality of this situation applies. This raises the question of Aloe's potential role in treating the aftermath of chronic and degenerative illness. Once the causes of chronic destruction have been removed, what is left is a lesion, just much as when the body is injured through trauma. The causes of chronicity will always have to be removed before healing can occur, and for that to be achieved, the causes of chronicity itself have to be understood. That is a prerequisite. We shall be examining the role of the healing process in that type of situation, as well as just in the healing of wounds.

## Thermal and Radiation Burns

Several papers and communications have confirmed that the condition of burns improves by treatment with Aloe. There was a very early report on this by Crewe (1939) "Aloes in the treatment of burns and scalds". Cera and colleagues (1980) wrote a report entitled "The therapeutic efficacy of Aloe cream in thermal injuries" and "The therapeutic efficacy of Aloe in thermal injuries: two case reports". Rodriguez-Bigas (1988) wrote "Comparative evaluation of *Aloe vera* in the management of burn wounds in guinea pigs." Kaufman (1989) wrote "*Aloe vera* and burn wound healing." All these papers and many more assert the impressive efficacy of Aloe in relieving the inflammation of burns and/or helping them to heal. On the subject of radiation burns, many papers have been published, beginning with Collins & Collins (1935), who wrote "Roentgen dermatitis treated with fresh whole leaf of *Aloe vera*", up to Stepanova (1977) "Chemical composition and biological activity of dry Aloe leaves". Without making any special effort to be comprehensive, the author easily found 14 papers asserting Aloe's effectiveness for radiation burns and 10 for thermal burns. These positive conclusions about the action of Aloe really cannot be faulted at all.

## Leg Ulcers and Dermatoses

A paper by Zawahry *et al* (1973) of Cairo reported some very successful treatments of leg ulcers with *Aloe vera* gel in three patients. This is only a clinical report, not an organized trial, and this author has found no other report of the subject of leg ulcer treatment. The fact that the results were so very favorable is really most impressive. As the above authors state, "Chronic leg ulcers usually have proved resistant to treatment, a handicap for the patient and a challenge for the doctor. Therefore, the introduction of a rapid and efficient healing agent would be a great advance." The ability of Aloe to promote healing is clearly the paramount effect here and it really is not obvious why these author's findings have not been taken up by others. The known properties of Aloe make it ideally suited to this purpose. Probably, subject to some properly organized trials, this could become a virtually standard treatment for leg ulcers and so relieve much suffering.

The same authors also obtained very positive results with *Aloe vera* in cases of seborrhoea, acne and alopecia. Again, these are very limited clinical observations, but the results given are clearly positive and very interesting. In particular, the report by these authors that *Aloe vera* can stimulate hair growth should certainly be further investigated, just in case *Aloe vera* could provide what has been so long wanted, an effective hair restorer. The report actually states that one bald man actually regrew some hair, not a very impressive amount. But some, while those with a serious, though lesser hair loss problem progressed very well.

Other authors had previously studied Aloe in relation to skin conditions. Dermatitis in dogs had been investigated in several papers and found to be helped very significantly. However, early studies by Crewe (1939) had related to burns and had used the aloin fraction. Anton & Haag-Berrurier (1980) also discuss the use of anthrainones from various plant sources in the treatment of conditions such as psoriasis. The usefulness of gel in psoriasis or related conditions does not appear to have been clearly established, and if Aloe has efficacy at all in that connection, this may be due to the aloin fraction or residual traces of it. This suggests at least the possibility that skin conditions, if treated with either Aloe gel or whole leaf extract, should perhaps be supplemented with a modest proportion of the aloin fraction. The paper by Zawahry and colleagues (1973) still appears to stand as the most interesting and, indeed, promising publication about Aloe in skin disease, as opposed to its use on externally damaged skin.

## Diabetes

The likely basis for Aloe's favorable action on diabetic problems was discussed in chapter 6. The probability of Aloe helping patients appears to be high because animal work has demonstrated a hypoglycemic effect (i.e. a blood sugar reducing effect when blood sugar is too high) and because actions which Aloe has been proven to exert are almost bound to be helpful with the side-effects and complications of diabetes. Therefore, we are here just concerned with the literature which has been published and to what extent it indicates that a favorable action is likely or possible.

This author has found just one paper which reports the effects of Aloe on human diabetics. This is by Ghannam *et al* (1986) from workers in Riyadh, Saudi Arabia. Their abstract makes the interesting statement that "The dried sap of the Aloe plant (aloes) is one of several traditional remedies used for diabetes in the Arabian peninsula." The study concerned five patients only, who all had non-insulin-dependent diabetes (NIDD). Two of these patients yielded two separate sets of experimental data, making seven records in all. Although the sample of patients is so small, the results obtained were most impressive. The fasting serum glucose levels were reduced from a mean of 273mg/dl before treatment to a mean of 151mg/dl after treatment. The insulin levels of these patients were unchanged. Interestingly, insulin levels in the blood of patients with NIDD commonly do not exhibit insulin deficiency and it appears that their problem has most to do with a relative insensitivity of the body tissues towards being influenced insulin. The inference here is that treatment with aloes in some manner not yet understood, improves the responsiveness of the body tissues towards insulin, making the insulin which is already circulating in the blood, more effective. In four out of the seven records, the patient's serum glucose fell to normal (80-100mg/dl) or just above that range, while in three other cases, although serum glucose was dramatically reduced, the level continued to hover at or just slightly above the renal threshold of 180mg/dl.

This paper is enormously encouraging towards the idea that aloes are an effective remedy against NIDD. Without a doubt more trials, and, in particular, are larger trial, preferably organized on a double-blind basis, are needed to clearly establish aloes as an effective remedy. This matter should not be left in abeyance because of its potential importance. The extent of the reduction in the blood sugar levels of these patients is both great and significant. Indeed, with the blood sugar reduced to 151mg/dl, the level has been reduced below the threshold at which sugar is obligatorily excreted into the urine. In that sense, these patients, after treatment, were not really diabetic at all, even though they still had a degree of hyperglycaemia. However, some surprise arises because the source of Aloe material being used was "bitter aloes", otherwise known as "drug aloes", and these names represent the aloin fraction. Therefore, if the Aloe material used is, indeed, effective against NIDD, then which subfraction of the aloin fraction is responsible? We do not know. Indeed, one cannot be completely sure that the effect is caused by an anthraquinone or phenolic component at all, since the sap of the plant, otherwise called the exudate, while it is a concentrate of anthraquinones and phenolics, also contains some of the same components which are in the gel or de-aloinized whole leaf extract.

Some confusion exists in the above paper about dose levels. A *Pharmacopoeia* reference dose for producing a purgative effect is given as 100-300mg/day. The dose given in the study to the patients concerned was "half a teaspoon daily", which is much more than the 100-300mg. However, later the dose used is quoted as being "too small to produce diarrhea". It may be that the investigators were employing an Aloe preparation far less concentrated that the reference *Pharmacopoeia* material, but this point is not explained. Future trials will therefore have to proceed with some care with regard to the type of preparation and the dose levels.

Ghannam and colleagues (1986) also studied the effect of Aloe treatment upon diabetic mice and reported an improvement (hypogly-cemic effect) of approximately 43% in their plasma glucose levels after 7 days of treatment. The remaining publications concerning Aloe and diabetes also deal with the treatment of animals. One such publication also comes from the Middle East, that of Farida and colleagues (1987) of Kuwait. They concluded that both Aloe, and another plant which they studied, myrrh, were significantly hypoglycemic and, by comparing the above study with their results from previous studies, also concluded that "different parts of the Aloe plant may lower blood glucose by different mechanisms". This holds the likelihood that an optimum Aloe product for the treatment of diabetes might need to contain, in addition to the material of the gel or whole leaf extract, some components from the aloin fraction. Therefore, the evidence is mounting that, for an Aloe product to be entirely optimized for the broadest possible spectrum of biomedical activities, the aloin fraction, or some parts of it, may, indeed, be needed. The work of Ghannam and colleagues (1986) also provides the result that Aloe exerts its hypoglycemic effect by reducing the body's production of blood glucose by the breakdown of protein (termed "gluconeogenisis"), whereas the positive action of myrrh in diabetes was achieved by increasing the tissue oxidation of glucose. The obvious inference from this is that Aloe, in a form which contains both main fractions, and myrrh, should be especially effective in combination for the treatment of diabetes.

## Peptic Ulcer

The specific subject of peptic ulcer is being addressed here partly to detail some Japanese work pertaining to the area and partly on account of work done by Blitz and colleagues in Florida (1963). In the latter study 12 patients with peptic ulcer were selected and *Aloe vera* gel was the sole source of treatment. It is notable that the gel was used because in the Japanese work components of the aloin fraction were recognized as being important. The twelve patients were "diagnosed clinically as having peptic ulcer, and having unmistakable roentgenographic evidence of duodenal cap lesions". The results of the Blitz work are summarized as "All of these patients had recovered completely by the end of 1961, so that at this writing at least 1 year has elapsed since the last treatment". Also "Clinically, *Aloe vera* gel has dissipated all symptoms" and "*Aloe vera* gel provided complete recovery". This is rather like the situation with regard to diabetes except that the trial was just slightly bigger. It is, indeed, tantalizing when one has only a small quantity of good information on such an important subject. The chances are that the misery of thousands of peptic ulcer sufferers could be removed through *Aloe vera*, but no one has proved it to the satisfaction of the medical profession. The pharmaceutical companies will not finance such trials because they can neither fully define the product as a drug, nor can they patent a herbal remedy so as to exclude other companies from the market. These are prime factors which are so far limiting the usage of Aloe in medicine; the lucky members of the public are the ones who know about it.

The Japanese work, done between 1970 and 1978, is significant insofar as it identifies in several papers that two factors in Aloe which diminish stomach secretion are aloenin and aloe-ulcin. They obtained these from *Aloe arborescens*. Aloenin is one of the individual components of the aloin fraction. It was listed in the Table of aloin components in Chapter 4 and is a phenolic compound of the type called a "quinonoid phenylpyrone". The fact that aloenin has this property means that it would have an action not unlike that of a drug such as cimetidine, which has a huge usage as a chemical drug for the treatment of peptic ulcer by suppression of stomach secretion. It is to be hoped that the action of substances from the gel or whole leaf extract upon peptic ulcer will be found to be by a less crude and less suppressive mechanism, which, hopefully might have something to do with correcting the underlying causes of peptic ulcer. Nonetheless, the Japanese findings show that, once again, a component of the aloin fraction seems to have a synergistic effect (i.e. a mutually enhancing effect) with the action of the gel components, raising once again, the question of arranging for combined treatment with both, either in one and the same product, or in complementary products. As for aloe-ulcin, the Japanese identified it with magnesium lactate. It is, frankly, hard to become convinced by that part of the evidence, because there is so little magnesium in Aloe: it takes much more to have known physiological effects. Therefore, this author does not draw any firm conclusions about aloe-ulcin, but this need not affect, in any way, the overall conclusions in relation to peptic ulcer.

## Intestinal Conditions

One study in particular stands out so far as the action of *Aloe vera* on the digestive system is concerned. This is the one by Bland, "Effect of Orally Consumed *Aloe Vera* Juice on Gastrointestinal Function in Normal Humans" (1985). It is a really excellent study and report on the effects of *Aloe vera* juice on the digestive system. The factors studied are (1) gastric pH, (2) stool specific gravity, (3) protein digestion/absorption and (4) stool microbiology, (5) bowel flora putrefactive activity as determined by blood levels of indican, an amine by putrefactive bacteria from the amino acid tryptophan. All these factors appear to be changed positively by the treatment. This is another paper which, incidentally, makes a point about the dose of Aloe juice to be used. The dose used in the study is stated to be 6oz., i.e. 170ml, or approximately 1L of the juice every six days.

Bland found that urinary levels of indican were reduced after Aloe treatment (by one full unit). The amount of it that is excreted is inversely proportional to the efficiency of protein digestion and absorption. He found that stool specific gravity was reduced by an average of "0.37 units". This was interpreted as indicating "improved water holding characteristics of the stool and decreased bowel transit time" The pH measurements showed "a drop of 1.88 units" as a result of *Aloe vera* administration. It is clear that this pH movement is in the right direction. Also, six out of ten subjects in the study showed markedly better stool microbiology, most particularly in respect of a lower yeast count. The bacterial population of the intestines are a very important parameter, since the pathogens (disease-causing organisms) and the putrefactive bacteria thrive in, and also create, and alkaline environment (which means high pH). A bacterial population which is more consistent with good bowel health is a population of acid-producers. It is clear from the results reported by Bland that the *Aloe vera* is encouraging the multiplication and colonization in the bowel of these acid-producing types.

These are the principal conclusions of the Bland paper. The above observations which he reported are definitive and entirely favorable to the action of *Aloe vera*. However, he goes on to make quite a number of observations concerning problem gut conditions, and their interaction with wheat intake, their relationship to arthritis, and the formation of incomplete breakdown products of the food constituents, which then spark off immune damaging responses and inflammatory conditions. Obviously, more such studies are badly needed. These further observations reported by Bland, which are summarized below, serve to show the nature and causes of these adverse gut conditions. Because they involve the immune system and are also, in many cases, inflammatory, it is obvious from the knowledge we have that *Aloe vera* is very likely to help

Bland makes reference to *Aloe vera* having been found helpful in the past "in the management of various food allergic symptoms or arthritis-like pain". It is known from the work of Dr. Hemmings, whom he quotes, that incomplete protein breakdown products from such reactive foods as gluten from wheat or casein from milk can be transported through the "leaky" gastrointestinal mucosa into the systemic circulation. They then initiate either antibody-antigen reactions in systemic circulation which can aggravate the symptoms of arthritis. Alternatively they may participate in direct antigen assault upon the gastrointestinal mucosa increasing the risk of inflammatory bowel disorders.

Bland points out that some of these incomplete protein breakdown products may have chemical reactivity similar to that of the internal hormones called endorphins and, if absorbed into the systemic circulation, may actually initiate bowel biochemical changes associated with what has been called "brain allergy". When these incomplete protein breakdown products, through poor protein digestion/absorption, are delivered into the bloodstream  initiate antigen-antibody complexes. These complexes can be trapped in the liver or in joint spaces and initiate inflammatory processes that have the clinical manifestations of pain and edema. This may explain why Rasmussen and his colleagues have found that a dietary fast can be helpful in reducing the symptoms of rheumatoid arthritis in stricken patients. In these cases, absence of food intake for a time, may have resulted in a decreased load of incomplete breakdown  products in the blood.

Recently, it has been found that in individuals who suffer from coeliac disease, that wheat protein contains a dietary antigen, alpha gliadin, which can activate T-suppressor cell activity and reduce the body's immunity. This may account for why coeliac disease is often associated with the symptoms of inflammatory bowel disease. Non-steroidal anti-inflammatory drugs commonly used to treat arthritis, actually increase the permeability of the gut to antigens and may increase the antigen-antibody complex formation and increase the long-term progression of the disease. It is also known that alcohol abuse can lead to a "leaky" gut with increasing risk of exposure to dietary antigens.

From this it is possible to conclude that, firstly, Bland himself has clearly demonstrated a number of very favorable effects of *Aloe vera* upon the digestive system taken as a whole, many of which are particularly likely to affect bowel health either directly or indirectly. Secondly, the possibilities for the use of *Aloe vera* for the digestive system are probably much greater even than Bland's own experiments have demonstrated. This author's comments and suggestions about the fundamental causes of adverse bowel conditions, certainly point the way towards and expanded application for *Aloe vera*, both for the maintenance of digestive health and also across a very broad spectrum of gastrointestinal medicine. This is a conclusion which, as has been mentioned already, has been largely anticipated by alternative and complementary medical practitioners and their patients, who see no reason to wait for fully documented orthodox medical evidence.

## Benign and Malignant Tumors

There appear to have been no human trials organized to discover whether or not *Aloe vera* is effective or supportive in cancer therapy. Therefore, the evidence we have is of a lesser kind. At this stage it would, indeed, be grossly irresponsible of anyone to offer *Aloe vera* as an effective cancer treatment, or, even worse, as *the cure* for cancer. Nonetheless, the indications that are available from the literature, showing that *Aloe vera* has an anti-cancer effect, either upon cells in tissue culture, or in the living animal, are most impressive. Of course, effectiveness in animals cannot be safely extrapolated to effectiveness in human cases. It is amazing, however, that in view of all the positive indications which exist for the anti-cancer effects of *Aloe vera* that no medical studies have been initiated in human cancer.

The immune system is, of course, the system which must tackle the job of ridding the body of tumors. It is considered very probable that most people throw up malignant cells in their body during their lifetime, perhaps they do so many times. The reason that cancer does not develop is that the immune system defenses are alert enough to deal with the abnormal cells and eliminate them. Cancer apparently, only develops when the immune system is sufficiently compromised to allow the abnormal cells to grow. The profound positive effect of Aloe on the immune system has already been fully discussed. We begin, therefore, from a very positive aspect, that it is inherently likely that an agent which galvanizes the immune system so successfully against bacteria, viruses and fungi, will also have a certain strengthening and encouraging effect when it comes to tumors.

The first definite reference to an anti-cancer effect of Aloe which this author has found is dated 1969 in a paper by Soeda of Japan. There was a further such reference by other authors from Japan in 1972. These were reports on the use of Aloe to treat animals with tumors, and showed that the tumors were inhibited. This type of work continued to be carried out by Japanese workers. Papers appeared by Yagi and colleagues (1977), Suzuki (1979), Imanishi and colleagues (1981), Yoshimoto and colleagues (1987) and Imanishi (1993). This work all concerned animal tumors and was carried out either by treating animals that were carrying tumors and demonstrating inhibition of the tumors, or by studying the immunological aspects of the problem, for example, by looking at the activation of the animals T-lymphocytes of the type which would have the job of tackling the tumor cells. Some of these papers were primarily concerned with isolating and studying fractions of the polysaccharide from Aloe and finding out which ones exhibited anti-tumor effects. One interesting aspect of the above is that the work of Soeda (1969) was carried out using Cape aloes (*Aloe ferox*) and preparations of Cape aloes usually contain the aloin fraction. Much of the other work used *Aloe arborescens*. This species is said not to have a separate section of the leaf which is removable as "gel", so the work with *Aloe arborescens* is generally carried out with whole leaf extracts. Where whole leaf extracts have been used as such, there is once again room for speculation that components of the aloin fraction may have some contributory role in the biomedical activity. However, very often the material used in the studies was a separated fraction isolated from an original whole leaf extract and composed either of polysac-charide or glycoprotein. In these cases it is more probable that the aloin components were largely or wholly removed and that the activity resided in these higher molecular weight biomolecules.

There is also some tissue culture work done in the USA by Winters and colleagues (1981). In this work, fractions of extracts of fresh leaves and commercially "stabilized" *Aloe vera* gel were obtained which contained high levels of polysaccharide or glycoprotein. Substances in fluid fractions from these extracts were found to markedly promote attachment and growth of human normal, but not tumor, cells and to enhance healing of wounded cell monolayers. This experiment is, perhaps, far from the *in vivo* condition, but it may be interpreted that the activities of normal cells were being enhanced by the *Aloe vera*, but not those of the tumor cells, a condition which should favor the eventual predominance of normal cells.

The state of these investigations, lacking human trials, leaves one simply failing to understand why favorable laboratory studies have not been followed up with any form of clinical trial. This author would unhesitatingly use *Aloe vera* in cases of cancer where the patient was seeking a way back to normal health by natural means. This is because he takes the view that where a particular biomedical activity has been demonstrated, and where the agent concerned is definitely completely harmless and many beneficial effects have been shown, then it is in the patient's interest to use the substance. He sees no need to wait for a formal proof of benefit for the particular disease state. After all, the fully confirmed information which we undoubtedly possess about *Aloe vera* shows it to be a most potent biomedical agent which is without doubt good for the patient, whatever it may or may not do for a particular named disease. Medical practitioners are there, first and foremost, to take actions to benefit patients.

The book by Lee Ritter *"Aloe vera* - A Mission Discovered" (1993) takes a more bullish view of the situation regarding *Aloe vera* and cancer, reporting one case of a "cure" in a patient who had 17 liver tumors and was cured and another who had breast cancer and who was "cured" by means of *Aloe vera*. The present author does not necessarily disbelieve the truth of these statements or the fact that the cures occurred, but the reiteration of such curative incidents does nothing to establish the role of Aloe in the minds of the skeptical. These reports will always be dismissed as anecdotal, however many of them there are, and they do not even begin to substitute for properly organized clinical trials.

No papers have been found dealing specifically with benign tumors and Aloe, but many of the same principles would be expected to apply as with malignant tumors.

## Arthritis

In view of the prevalence of arthritis it is surprising that we have so little information about the role of Aloe in patients with this complaint. The observations of Bland given above within this Chapter, are valuable in this connection. A study of the available literature has little to add to what was said about Aloe and arthritis in Chapter 6. Also Mad's Laboratories, Inc., (1984), list arthritis as one of the conditions benefiting from *Aloe vera* gel in *The Ageless Beauty Ingredient*, 9th Edition (South Hackensack, New Jersey). There are strong *a priori* reasons why one would anticipate a noteworthy improvement from the use of Aloe, based just on the nature of the fundamental actions of Aloe and the nature of arthritis as a disease. However, clinical studies are mostly lacking. Work by Davis and co-workers, of the Pennsylvania College of

Podiatric Medicine, Philadelphia, U.S.A. (1985-86) has provided some positive results, but used either anthraquinones from Aloe, or whole homogenized Aloe, demonstrating anti-arthritic effect. Hence, in both these papers, aloin fraction was either the medicine used, or the entire leaf, containing the aloin fraction, was present. Hence, once again, the prospect that individual components of the aloin fraction may be needed for some of Aloe's bioedical properties, raises its head. It is an issue which will require full consideration. Hence, such evidence that we have certainly contains the strong suggestion of a role for Aloe in arthritis, but the presence of these aloin-type components may, indeed, be required.

*Eleven*

# HOW ALOE MAY INFLUENCE
# INFLAMMATION AND HEALING

This section brings together the knowledge already explained about Aloe's composition, effects on diseases and symptoms. It looks at the effects which Aloe has upon cells apart from immune stimulation, and concentrates upon understanding, so far as possible, the anti-inflammatory and cell-multiplying, (or healing effects) of Aloe.

## Anti-Inflammatory Action

The anti-inflammatory action of Aloe is one of the best-known actions. It is clearly responsible for all the early benefits from applying Aloe gel, and various preparations and ointments and creams of Aloe to wounds, cuts and abrasions of all kinds. It must also be responsible for the early benefits in sports injuries, frost-bite, burns and radiation burns, in the tissue-damage applications associated with dentistry and otolaryngology, as well as its earliest effects upon arthritis and upon infections. Many kinds of beneficial action which Aloe has been noted to have upon other conditions which are primarily inflammatory in nature, would also be examples of this same basis of action, including insect bites and stings of all kinds and also jelly-fish stings. Much skin disease also is associated with a lot of inflammation, and clearly benefits from the same action. It is certainly reasonable to list the anti-inflammatory action as being one of the fundamental beneficial actions of Aloe, and as one of those actions which has favorable knock-on consequences.

Quite a significant number of papers have been published which clearly report that *Aloe vera*, or other Aloe, has a notable anti-inflammatory effect. For example, "Tissue response to Aloe vera gel following periodontal surgery", by Payne in 1970, "Topical anti-inflammatory activity of *Aloe vera* as measured by ear swelling." by Davis, Leitner & Russo, 1987, "Processed *Aloe vera* Administered Topically Inhibits Inflammation", by Davis, Roenthal, Cesario & Rouw, (1989) and "*Aloe vera* and the inflamed synovial pouch model." by Davis, Stewart & Bregman, 1992. However, there have by now been so many publications confirming anti-inflammatory activity that the existence of such activity is in no doubt whatever. The discussion which continues is about the mechanism of the anti-inflammatory effect and which chemical components of *Aloe vera* are involved in this.

## Steroids

Since it is well known that steroids exert an anti-inflammatory effect and are widely used for this in the form of steroid drugs, one theory was that the natural plant steroids which *Aloe vera* contains were capable of acting rather like steroid drugs. This was never a very attractive theory, since steroid drugs are known to alternative pactitioners as naturopathically suppressive, and all medical practitioners, both alternative and orthodox, recognize the very undesirable side-effects which steroids have. The idea that *Aloe vera* might work on inflammation only by virtue of the steroids which it contains, would certainly not be good for the image of *Aloe vera* in the eyes of those who embrace naturopathic and vitalistic principles. However, it was clearly necessary to find out the truth about this in an unbiased way. The most extensive and penetrating inquiries into this matter have been conducted by Dr. Robert H. Davis and his team of Pennsylvania. Several of their papers have inquired into the mechanism of anti-inflammatory effect. Of special importance is "*Aloe Vera*, Hydrocortisone and Sterol Influence on Wound Tensile Strength and Anti-inflammation." Davis, Didonato, Johnson, & Stewart, (1994). This paper highlights the fact that steroids exert their well-known anti-inflammatory effect at the expense of partially inhibiting the wound-healing powers of the tissues. This is very undesirable, since, whilst an anti-inflammatory effect is desirable in itself, another priority with regard to injuries or any open sore, is to initiate healing. Healing action is a different effect, since it depends upon securing the multiplication of those cell types which have the power to replace damaged, dead or excised tissues with new and which can give some physical strength to contribute to the closure of an open wound.

By contrast with this anti-inflammatory, yet anti-healing effect of steroid drugs, particularly that of the steroid drug hydrocortisone, *Aloe vera* was found to possess the special combination of being anti-inflammatory and yet pro-healing. The particular plant steroids that are present in *Aloe vera* are known. They are called Lupeol, (beta-sitosterol and campesterol. All three were confirmed to be topically anti-inflammatory in much the same way as steroid drugs. The authors proceeded to show that lupeol, (37.0%), (beta-sitosterol, (31.1%) and campesterol, (24.2%) all reduced inflammation. The dose-response curve for lupeol is similar to that of *Aloe vera* and "implies that sterols are definitely responsible for a portion of aloe's anti-inflammatory activity". The authors relate the relative anti-inflammatory activities of the three sterols of *Aloe vera* to their chemical formulae, pointing out especially their resemblance to hydrocortisone. They also demonstrated that Lupeol is inhibitory of wound healing in much the same way as hydrocortisone, and therefore cannot be responsible for the stimulatory effects of *Aloe vera* on wound-healing, which must come from other quite separate wound-healing stimulants. Therefore, whilst it is possible that the natural steroids of Aloe do exert a steroid-drug-like effect to some degree, this is not the principal or characteristic effect which Aloe has on sites of inflammation, because Aloe's effect certainly also stimulates healing. Moreover, Aloe contains other anti-inflammatory ingredients as well, not just the steroids, so the actual contribution made by steroids to Aloe's anti-inflammatory action could be quite small, but this has not yet been clearly quantified.

Then these authors consider by what mechanism these steroids exert their anti-inflammatory effect. They suggest that one way lies in their ability to depress cholesterol synthesis in the lymphocytes and elsewhere. "Cholesterol stimulates lymphocyte proliferation and granulocyte formation: two factors involved in the inflammatory response. Granulocytes are a large group of non-lymphocyte white cells. Therefore, reduced cholesterol synthesis caused by the steroid may be a key factor in decreasing inflammation by reducing lymphocyte proliferation and granulocyte formation". "Furthermore, cholesterol stimulates macrophages, which are largely responsible for appropriate lymphocytic activity. Consequently, sterols may lower inflammation by reducing cholesterol availability and decreasing lymphocyte activity."

Dr. Davis and colleagues also demonstrated that when the self-healing ability of wounded tissues was inhibited by the use of the steroid drug hydrocortisone, administration of Aloe reversed that inhibitory effect to an extent which was directly related to the dose of Aloe. Mice given 1mg per kg hydrocortisone showed a depression in wound-healing by hydrocortisone of 46.7%. From this depressed level the stimulation of woundhealing by *Aloe vera* was 66.7% at 100mg / kg of Aloe vera and 100% at 300mg / kg of *Aloe vera*. So, *Aloe vera* stimulated wound-healing in spite of treatment with hydrocortisone and, in the words of the authors, "therefore must contain powerful growth-promoting agents to show the effects that it did while also acting to reduce inflammation". We shall need to look more closely at these growth-promoting agents. These authors conclude that sterols in *Aloe vera* cannot be responsible for the wound-healing properties of the whole plant. *Aloe vera* contains numerous strong growthpromoting factors, quoted by these authors as being certain amino acids, gibberellin and indole-3-acetic acid "which the authors unpublished work indicates are probably most responsible for Aloe's wound healing property".

## Bradykininase

Again, these same authors also say that Aloe has the enzyme activity called bradykininase. Bradykinin is a peptide substance which causes increased vascular permeability to stimulate inflammation. Bradykininase breaks down bradykinin, reducing inflammation. Aloe possesses bradykininase activity and also decreases inflammation in this way. Other papers which confirm the presence of bradykininase enzyme in Aloe. These are "Bradykininase activity in Aloe extract" by Fujita., Teradaira, & Nagatsu, 1976, "Anti-Bradykinin Active Material in *Aloe saponaria*" by Yagi., Harada, Iwadare, & Nishioka, I., 1982 and "Bradykinin-Degrading Glycoprotein in *Aloe arborescens var. natalensis.*" by Yagi, A, Harada, N., Shimomura, K., & Nishioka, I. 1986.

## Prostaglandin Hormone Complex

Another important system controlling and affecting levels of inflammation is the prostaglandin complex of hormones in the body. Unlike the better known hormones, these are specialized hormones being produced and also exerting their effects upon the tissues that produce them, or, at least, tissues quite close by. The classes of prostaglandin hormones known as Series 2 prostaglandins are pro-inflammatory, i.e. they encourage, or accentuate, inflammation. Hence, any influence which tends to increase Series 2 prostaglandin production will tend to increase inflammation, while any influence which reduces Series 2 prostaglandin formation, will reduce inflammatory tendencies. Several papers have focused upon the ability of Aloe to influence the formation of prostaglandins, for example, "Anti-prostaglandins and anti-thromboxanes for treatment of frostbite" by Raine and colleagues (1980), "Inhibition of arachidonic acid oxidation *in vitro* by vehicle components", by Penneys, 1982, and "Prostaglandins and thromboxanes", Hegger & Robson, 1983. The arachidonic acid mentioned in the second of these papers is a fatty acid which converts into prostaglandins. This work does seem to establish that there is some anti-prostaglandin effect in Aloe, and that this probably does have a role to play in its very important anti-inflammatory action. It is not possible, however, on the basis of the evidence we have, to say, what proportion of the anti-inflammatory effect can be ascribed to (a) Natural steroids of Aloe and (b) Bradykininase enzyme or (c) Anti-prostaglandin effects of Aloe.

## Healing Action

It is necessary to turn now to the specific "healing" effects of Aloe. This is certainly a separate type of action from the anti-inflammatory effect. The latter effect, as we have seen, calls for the *inhibiting* of certain processes, such as cholesterol synthesis, the *inhibiting* of prostaglandin formation, or the *inhibiting* of bradykininase enzyme. By complete contrast with this, a healing action calls for the positive stimulation of those cells which grow and multiply to effect the formation and physical strengthening of wound tissues. The process of healing has more in common with the process of immune stimulation, since both are positive stimulatory processes, not inhibitory.

## Effect of Mannans

It is not surprising, therefore, that since these two processes of immune stimulation and healing have something in common, that they should also be linked in another way. Both seem to reside, at least in part, in the high molecular weight carbohydrate-rich fraction of Aloe. In chapter 9 it has been clearly shown how the immune stimulation effect is mediated through this fraction. That the healing action is also at least partly mediated through this fraction is clearly demonstrated in the published literature. For example, a paper by Tizard, Carpenter, & McAnalley, 1989, entitled "The Biological Activities of Mannans and related complex Carbohydrates", addresses itself more generally to the question of the biomedical effects of mannose-containing carbohydrates of this type, wherever they come from. The authors conclude that mannose containing products increase macrophage activity and promote wound-healing. Stimulation of macrophages will increase cell and tissue growth, fibroblast activity and fibroblast proliferation. Aloe, containing mannose, "may also promote wound-healing in this way".

The reader is reminded at this point that the stimulatory nature of the immune system effects were cited by J.C. Pittman in 1992 in a short review and summary entitled "Immune enhancing effects of Aloe", which was quoted in chapter 9. This quotation was "Acemannan has direct effects on the immune system, activating and stimulating macrophages, monocytes, antibodies and T-cells." The reader is reminded that Acemannan is a trade name which has been applied to the mannose-rich polysaccharide fraction from Aloe.

Davis and colleagues found that *Aloe vera* increases collagen (protein) and proteoglycan synthesis, and that this results in increased tissue repair without loss of anti-inflammatory activity. They suggested that the mechanism might be that mannose-6-phosphate fits the growth factor receptors on the surface of the fibroblasts, enhancing their activity. This paper is Davis, Didonato, & Hartman, "Anti-inflammatory and wound-healing activity of a growth substance in *Aloe vera*", 1994. This very mechanism has been illustrated already in chapter 9, showing a route to the stimulation of fibroblasts, cells which produce collagen (protein) fibers to strengthen the new tissue formations which heal wounds. Inherent within this idea is the concept that fibroblast cells, which are key cells in forming the structure of connective tissue, possess special receptors of the type discussed in chapter 8, which are sensitive to mannose-6-phosphate and hence to mannose-containing polysaccharides, mannose-containing glycoproteins, and breakdown products derived from these large mannose-rich molecules. Macrophages and other immune cells have similar surface receptors. This is reflected in a paper by Winters (1993), which was quoted already in chapter 9. After presenting experimental results, Winters declares "These results suggest that these Aloe lectins were active at alpha D-glucose and mannose sites and not at n-acetyl glucosamine sites". The white blood cells being used in this work appear to have been predominantly lymphocytes.

Hence, it appears that the "final common pathway" for initiating both the immune-stimulatory effect and the tissue-healing effect of Aloe, is the stimulation of predominantly mannose-sensitive cell-surface receptors. In the one case the cell-surface involved is that of immune system cells, and in the other it is the surface of the fibroblasts of connective tissues.

## Plant Growth Hormones

Prof. Davis considers that gibberellin (a plant growth hormone) in Aloe increases wound-healing by increasing protein synthesis. It has been said to do this by binding to a section of DNA and consequently affecting the copying of the DNA so as to make protein. The authors Davis, Didonato, & Hartman, in "Anti-inflammatory and wound-healing activity of a growth substance in *Aloe vera*", 1994, say that gibberellin, isolated from Aloe, increased wound-healing more than 100% in mice. Indole-3-acetic acid, an auxin, which is also a plant growth hormone, was also reported to increase protein synthesis by increasing uptake of amino acids. Little work directly upon gibberellin in Aloe appears to have been published, but one paper which mentions it specifically is "Aloe vera and gibberellin: anti-inflammatory activity in diabetes." by Davis & Maro, 1989. Some of the amino acids have also been referred to as growth-stimulants by Prof. Davis's group, but no definite role for these has yet been clarified, nor attributed with any certainty to any individual amino acids.

## Summary

From all the foregoing it can be seen that the phenomena of (a) anti-inflammatory effect and (b) healing action, are multi-factorial. That is to say, they are the result of a good many factors coming together and exerting their own distinct influences simultaneously, to produce the overall effects. The knowledge which has been gathered is impressive, though it falls short of complete explanation or complete understanding. Nonetheless, it serves to give a fair mental image of the types of processes that are going on when Aloe exerts its effects.

In the next Chapter we turn to consider that ways in which the three prime known actions of Aloe work in concert, not only with each other, but also with the known secondary effects of Aloe, to produce important beneficial effects upon chronic illness. It also becomes possible to address the question as to which medical conditions which have not yet been subjected to medical trials with Aloe, most stand to benefit, on theoretical and inferential grounds, from the future application of the therapeutic effects of Aloe.

*Twelve*

# HOW ALOE MAY INITIATE A CASCADE OF BENEFICIAL CHANGES AT CELLULAR LEVEL, WITH MULTIPLE CONSEQUENCES

This chapter is concerned with how one thing leads to another within the cell, within tissues and within the body to produce the observed benefits. We will be dealing here with strong hypotheses rather than fully established fact, but they should be mature and advanced hypotheses based directly upon the detail that is contained within the scientific research.

## Disease states likely to be helped through Aloe's Prime Actions

The foregoing chapters have shown that the therapeutic actions of Aloe can be divided, for the most part, into three categories, according which of the three prime actions of Aloe predominate in bringing them about. The following list details a great many of these cited therapeutic actions on named conditions, and allocates them according to whether the prime action of Aloe that is involved is (a) anti-inflammatory, (b) immunostimulant or (c) healing effect. In some cases more than one prime action is clearly involved. Even so, the list is not fully comprehensive, by any means, to cover all the medical conditions that have been claimed to have been helped by Aloe.

## Inflammation

Wounds, thermal burns, frost-bite, radiation burns, sports injuries, skin disease, pain, dental applications, otolaryngeal applications, hepatitis, peptic ulcer, leg ulcers, diabetes, arthritis, inflammatory digestive system complaints e.g. intestinal, insect stings, jelly-fish stings, post surgical uses, psoriasis, eczema, bursitis, tendonitis, gingivitis, sunburn, lupus erythematosus, gout, complications of diabetes, myositis (prolonged muscle inflammations), dandruff, sprains and strains.

## Immunostimulant

Antibacterial, anti-viral, anti-fungal, arthritis, wounds and burns, hepatitis, digestive system complaints e.g. intestinal, Type I diabetes, hepatitis, skin disease, tumors, immuno-depressive conditions (Epstein-Barr virus, Chronic Fatigue Syndrome, systemic candidiasis, HIV infection and others), acne, herpes simplex, athlete's foot, warts, including vaginal warts, respiratory infections, vaginitis, pruritis ani, pruritis valvae, leg ulcers, malignancies

## Healing action

Mouth ulcers, chemical burns, wounds, thermal burns, radiation burns, sports injuries, skin disease, dental applications, otolaryngeal applications, peptic ulcer, leg ulcers, diabetes, arthritis, digestive system complaints e.g. intestinal, post surgical uses, psoriasis, eczema, bursitis, tendonitis, gingivitis, sunburn, lupus erythematosus, gout, respiratory infections.

## Other, Miscellaneous or uncertain

Corns, calluses, in-grown toe-nails, muscle spasms, leg cramps, hypoglycemic effect in Type II diabetes.

## Overlaps between the Prime Actions

There are, of course, some overlaps between the main actions. For example, the "healing action" is the same thing as causing a growth of new tissue, and that involves stimulating cell division. Stimulation of cell division is often referred to as the "mitogenic effect". It takes place within the immune system as well as in the connective tissues which heal wounds. Naturally, when this "mitogenic action" succeeds in increasing the numbers of immune system cells which are available for the body's defenses, it has, in effect, produced a fortification of the immune system. In such a case, it has done so, not by stimulating the existing immune cells to increase their activities, but simply by providing a greater number of immune cells.

Another way in which an overlap of this sort occurs is when the active substances of Aloe stimulate the macrophages of the immune system and the macrophages, in turn, secrete substances which stimulate and accelerate healing. A paper of Prof. Davis and co-workers in 1994 stresses that macrophages play an important role in decreasing long-term inflammation and stimulate fibroblasts to increase wound healing. In this connection they quote a review of the role of macrophages in wound repair by DieGelmann, Cohen, & Kaplan, 1981 as well as two basic texts of medicine and physiology. This role of macrophages is quite well known and well recognized. Prof. Davis's group also quote that "They (macrophages) undergo phagocytosis-induced secretion of interleukin-1 and tumor necrosis factor, stimulating fibroblast activity". The two special immune system biochemicals mentioned are very important messenger substances acting from or between immune system cells. For example, both the interleukins and tumor necrosis factor are involved in body's defense mechanisms against tumors. In this instance they are cited as "stimulating fibroblast activity", which means stimulating healing. So, an action by Aloe substances, which started out as an action upon the immune system, and which does in fact have and immuno-stimulant result, ends up also having the additional effect of encouraging healing.

This means that even with the three prime actions of Aloe which have been identified in this book, there is a certain interconnectedness between them. In the above example, a substance within Aloe which directly increases one of these actions, ends up indirectly increasing one of the others.

## Diagrammatic Plot of the Pattern of Aloe's Actions

We now look at the different actions of Aloe in the form of a diagram which helps to understand the relationships between them. This diagram in figure summarizes the sequences of events which lead to the three prime actions of Aloe. The hypoglycemic (anti-diabetic effect is also included within this diagram. The reader is asked to please trace the pathways involved in generating these actions as follows.

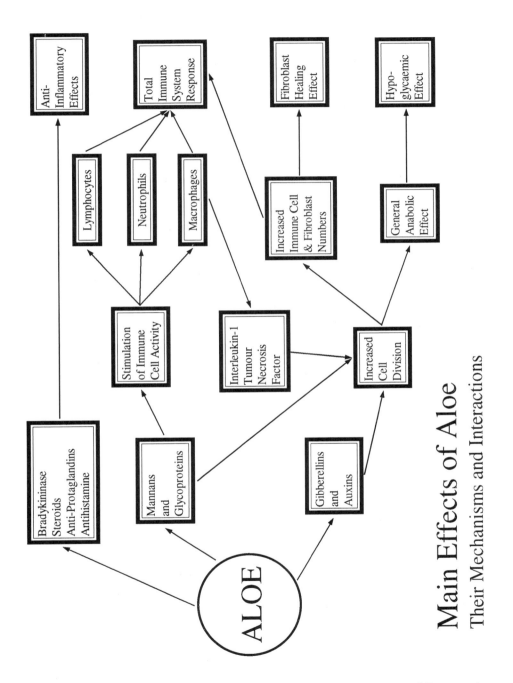

Figure 11. Main Effects of Aloe - Their Mechanisms and Interactions

1.   Bradykininase, steroids and anti-prostaglandin substances in Aloe lead to the overall anti-inflammatory effect. As anti-histamine action by components of Aloe has also been mooted in some literature, that too has been included. This pathway of events is represented along the top horizontal pathway in the diagram.

2.   The main high molecular weight, polysaccharide rich fraction of Aloe, which is a mixture of mannans (i.e. mannose polysac-charides) and glycoproteins, stimulates cell activity by interacting with cell-surface receptors as has been explained earlier. This effect influences the cells of the immune system, but specifically, lymphocytes, neutrophils and macrophages. This result, combined with the effects of increased cell numbers, which result from Aloe's mitogenic effect, give us the totality of the overall immune response to Aloe. This sequence is followed through in the central horizontal path on the diagram.

3.   At the same time plant growth factors, named gibberellins and auxins, together with the mannose-rich mannans and glycoproteins stimulate a variety of cell types to divide. It is clear that a number of immune cell types are included within that effect and also the fibroblasts, which give rise to the healing response within damaged tissues. The result of this cell division, of course, is increased cell numbers, within the immune system and also among the fibroblasts. The increased numbers of immune cells make their contribution to the overall immune response whilst the increases in the numbers of fibroblasts bring about the healing response in damaged tissues. This sequence is followed through in one of the lower horizontal paths on the diagram.

4.   As has been recounted already, the macrophages, upon being stimulated in their activities by mannans and glycoproteins, release two chemical messengers called interleukin-1 and tumor necrosis factor, and thereby further increasing the division and activity of other cells, including the fibroblasts which are responsible for healing. This is believed to have the end-result of enhancing the healing effect. This sub-pathway is traceable through the backward-directed arrows in the lower central part of the diagram.

5.   As an additional effect, the hypoglycemic effect has also been included, although its mechanism is less certain. It is worth noting, however, that increasing cell division calls for increasing synthesis of cell constituents to form these new cells. It therefore implies that

metabolism is being strongly directed, under the influence of Aloe, to synthetic activity rather than breakdown activity. The synthesis of cell constituents, leading their accumulation, is known as "anabolism" or an "anabolic effect". The opposite effect, that of encouraging break-down of cellular constituents, would be called catabolic. It would seem, therefore, that the general tendency of cells acting under the influence of Aloe is towards anabolism. Not only does cell division absolutely require this, but it is also a known metabolic influence of gibberellins to encourage protein synthesis, and hence, encourage the build-up of cellular material. Moreover, the receptor on the fibroblasts which unites with mannan, is one which also accepts the iinsulin-like growth factor. Insulin in an abundantly anabolic hormone, which again, accentuates Aloe's connection with anabolic, rather than catabolic effects. The inference which may be drawn from this, at least tentatively, is that the general nature of Aloe's effects are anabolic. This general tendency could well be at the route of the inhibition of gluconeogenesis by Aloe, which has been reported as being the way in which Aloe lowers the blood sugar of hyperglycemic individuals. This probable mechanism is represented in the bottom right hand part of the diagram.

This, then is the "Cascade" of processes which seems to lie at the basis of Aloe's total action. After these steps have occurred, the prime actions of Aloe represented in the diagram can start to influence medical conditions such as those listed out against the headings of "inflammation", "immunostimulant" and "healing action" at the start of this chapter. Influencing the health status of the patients in these conditions and reducing their symptoms therefore comes at the end of the cascade of events being described.

## The Holistic and Vitalistic Implications of Aloe's Actions

Up to this point in this book the actions of Aloe have been plotted in biochemical, physiological, immunological and pathological terms, in other words, according to the thinking and language of the medical sciences. However, Aloe's virtues appeal to a great many people who do not necessarily subscribe to all the precepts of orthodox medicine. These people are likely to say that they use Aloe "for its cleansing action", or for its "revitalizing effects" How is it possible that Aloe, as well as doing all that has been described in terms of medical and cellular effects that have been observed and studied by medical scientists, can also accomplish these less well defined functions that carry weight within alternative and complementary medicine. This author does consider that these things are mutually compatible.

So far as "cleansing" is concerned, this is generally understood to be the process of clearing out both metabolic waste products and environmental toxins that have entered the body and been taken up by its cells. Toxins produced by intestinal bacteria and then absorbed, also have a part to play.

The hypothesis that lies behind the concept of cleansing is, briefly, as follows. In naturopathic terms, the factor which most compromises bodily health is the accumulation of toxic waste and poisons in the living cell. The mechanism by which these substances produced their effects could never be specified by the early naturopaths. It is now clear, however, that what lay at the foundation of their mental concepts about this was the inhibition of cell enzymes, especially those which break down foods to yield energy, those which synthesize proteins, including the enzymes themselves, those concerned in the synthesis and maintenance of the nucleic acids, and those concerned with the formation and maintenance of the external and internal cellular membranes. These are the parts of the living processes of the cell which are the most vulnerable to damage by toxins. All such damage contributes to making the cell inefficient and ineffective where the cell was vital and active before. Cells become moribund and die under the influence of toxins. The event of cell death is preceded by a time when the cell is hypoactive (i.e. underactive) on account of its load of toxins. Most particularly the energy-generating mechanisms of the cell are damaged or hindered. The cell has less energy to work with. Its processes are slowed, its respiration, its synthesis of proteins, its ability to repair itself and replace its parts, and, most important, its ability to maintain its own internal environment, with the correct concentrations of sodium and potassium, calcium and magnesium. These are the processes of chronicity. It is a process which leads the body towards lowered vitality and activity.

In the naturopathic philosophy, onward progression of toxicity and of the chronic condition is a general disease-encouraging process. Some types of toxin affect one or more tissues or organs preferentially. In other cases the toxic effect is non-specific as to tissue type. The body organ or system fails and hence what disease develops then depends upon constitutional and inherited factors that are peculiar to each individual. It does mean, however, that it is generally true that the chronic diseases can be avoided by avoiding getting into toxic and chronic conditions.

*Aloe vera*, as we have seen, activates the immune cells, and in particular, it activates the scavenging macrophages and neutrophils which carry out clean-up operations. This role of the immune system makes it a great detoxifier. Those of them which operate within the confines of the lymphatic system, in the lymph glands, actually engage in cleaning up the lymph as it flows from the tissue drainage areas towards re-entry into the blood-stream. Aloe, as we have seen, also activates cells into a growth and replication phase, accompanied by much protein synthesis and the general build-up of tissue constituents. This is what has been termed "anabolism". Cells in this positively activated, constructive and reproductive phase have increased activity and this is emphasized by their increased oxygen consumption. Such activated cells have heightened metabolism and have moved far from the chronic state. It is therefore a fair interpretation of the actions of Aloe that it moves cells away from hypo-active and therefore chronic conditions towards the highly active states in which detoxification occurs readily due to the cell's favorable energy supply. Returning again for a moment to the condition of the immune system, it is a matter of clinical observation that patients with good and active immune systems are generally active healthy people, while low states of the immune system make for patients with unaccountable low energy, liable to all manner of pathologies and symptoms, perhaps veering towards a highly fatigued syndrome.

Seen in this way, provided one can perceive something, at least, of the naturopathic vision of what makes the human organism "tick", Aloe emerges as a kind of pick-me-up tonic. Not a tonic, or semi-panacea, based upon hype and over-imagination, but a "pick-me-up" tonic which has undergone much detailed scientific evaluation. The concept of a "tonic" is an old idea and the term is not much used today. This is because the idea of a medicine which would boost you whatever was wrong, which would build you up generally, has come to be thought of and an out-of-date and out-moded idea. The intricate knowledge about the mode of action of modern drugs, seemed to deny even the poss-ibility that there could be such a substance. However, this particular medical scientist has come to the conclusion that Aloe is, indeed, just this kind of a substance and medicine. And that conclusion is based upon the knowledge of the anti-inflammatory, immuno-stimulant and cell growth and replication (healing) activities of *Aloe vera*, all of which lead to its abilities to cleanse, detoxify, heal and repair. These activities together amount to a revitalizing influence.

## The/Illnesses, not covered by the Literature, for which *Aloe vera* should be tried

There now follows a note about a number of diseases in which part of the complaint is connected with immune systems troubles and/or inflammation. Literature about the application of Aloe to such diseases is wholly lacking or almost so. Yet, due to the nature of the diseases selected below, there is reason to be hopeful that a medicine with Aloe's spectrum of activities should be distinctly helpful. This list is by no means comprehensive - there are no doubt many more diseases which could be put into the same category.

## Multiple Sclerosis

This is a well known serious complaint of the nervous system. Nervous system function is adversely affected in many ways as the disease advances, resulting, in particular in ataxia (inability or difficulty in walking and other movements), loss of speech and other disabilities. Multiple sclerosis involves a component of autoimmunity, i.e. as explained in a previous chapter, the cells of the nervous tissue are damaged by an immune attack from the patient's own immune system, and it is certainly also an inflammatory condition. On these two counts, it would appear, on theoretical grounds at least, that multiple sclerosis is well placed to benefit from Aloe's known actions.

## Type I Diabetes - especially during the developmental stage

Quite apart from the hypoglycemic effect of Aloe, which is directly helpful with the control of the high blood sugar situation in diabetes, the anti-inflammatory effect of Aloe would be highly relevant in the developmental stages of Type I diabetes, when, once again, there is an autoimmune attack by the patient's own immune system upon the Islets of Langerhans in the pancreas. This early condition of the disease, which is referred to as "Islitis" or "Insulitis", consists of an inflamed condition of the Islets, due this immune attack. Aloe would appear to have the potential to both relieve the inflammation but also to improve the condition of the immune system so as to reduce or eliminate the immune attack which causes the problem.

## Crohn's Disease

This is a condition which affects the intestines, very often the small intestine. It involves much inflammation and malfunction of the intestines. It is possible that it may be associated with poor functioning of the immune elements within the intestinal wall. Since it is a condition much affected by wheat and other important allergens, it is likely that improvement of immune function in these cases would be helpful.

## Hyperthyroidism - Grave's Disease

The inclusion of hyperthyroidism here is, admittedly, speculative. However, there does appear to be a relationship between the inflammatory state - which is a state of high activity - and any state of hyperactivity. This is a relationship which will probably not be readily apparent to anyone schooled mainly in orthodox medical sciences, but it is one which is drawn out strongly by the study of Iridology - which consists of diagnosis from the iris of the eye. Iris diagnosis delivers information in naturopathic rather than in orthodox medical terms. And it shows inflammatory conditions and hyperactive conditions as being fundamentally similar. On this basis it can be speculated that the anti-inflammatory actions of Aloe may contribute to calming the over-activity of hyperthyroidism. Another reason for considering the treatment of hyperthryoidism with Aloe is that there is also an autoimmune contribution to the causation of hyperthyoidism.

## Allergic States

Allergies are an extremely common form of complaint today, often taking the form of multiple susceptibilities to different allergens, both food and non-food. They arise from a combination of factors, which may include the abuse of cow's milk by using it as a constant food source for very young babies and also the incidence of gastroenteritis in babyhood. Later in life, the poor conditions of the intestinal walls due to dietary and nutritional factors looms large, as does the role of antibiotics in damaging the integrity of the reticulo-endothelial system of the liver, and thereby exposing the immune system to incompletely digested food substances coming from the intestines. Exposure to toxicity and under-nutrition with micro-nutrients also make a most important contribution to the causes of allergic states, as also does the too frequent repetition of particular foods in the diet. All these factors taken together, have been leading to an epidemic of increasing serious allergic states within the populations of western countries.

In view of the position of allergies as diseases of the immune system, and the role of the reticulo-endothelial system of the liver in protecting the immune system, the known actions of Aloe with regard to the immune system would be expected to give Aloe a most positive potential role in the treatment of allergies.

## Liver Disease and Underfunction

One paper which reports positive action of Aloe on hepatitis, may simply have been reflecting the anti-viral effect of Aloe, mediated through the improvement of the immune system. However, two other reports, one which shows how Aloe can help with cirrhosis of the liver, and another which shows that Aloe can strongly support regeneration of the damaged liver (healing effect), at least give pointers to a possible role for Aloe in the treatment of either liver damage or chronic liver disease. This is definitely an area within which some real efforts with regard to clinical trials would be fully justified.

*Thirteen*

# HOW TO USE ALOE

## The User's Thinking which lies behind Treatment with Aloe

Readers who have assimilated the contents of chapters 1-12 will by this time have abundant reasons for regarding Aloe with a great deal of respect as a powerful herbal remedy with multifaceted potency within the widest field of "healing". At the same time many readers may have been quite properly impressed with Aloe's powers in specific healing directions, such as those applying to those named medical conditions which have been subjected to trials with Aloe for potential therapeutic application. For yet other people, who perhaps suffer from no illness or significant symptoms, the attraction of Aloe may well be its potential for maintaining good health by a general "toning up" effect, which is inherent in Aloe's fundamental actions, especially those having to do with maintaining or improving the condition of the immune system and increasing the oxygen consumption, and therefore the activity levels, within the tissues. These, effects, most emphatically, appear to offer a very positive route to the avoidance of the partially de-oxygenated, low-activity and toxic condition which is recognized, naturopathically and vitalistically, as constituting the state of "chronicity". Furthermore, while this state of "chronicity" is the major predisposing factor towards chronic illness, it does not yet form part of the philosophy and outlook of mainstream medicine. The concept is nonetheless wholly compatible with the principles of modern medical biochemistry.

It will be clear why it is that Aloe gets dubbed with emotive terms such as "The Silent Healer" and even "Panacea". This happens, even among quite well informed users of Aloe, not just people who are greatly influenced by hype and imagination. It does so because the nature of the fundamental actions of Aloe are to improve the status of some vitally important systems of the body which affect many functions. In this way it improves, generally, the biochemical status, activity levels and metabolic and functional competence of cells. Obviously, any such influence will be a most positive factor in keeping the individual safer than they would otherwise be, from developing chronic diseases in general. The painstaking process, which no doubt will have to be gone through, of thoroughly testing Aloe in clinical trials against every known chronic disease, is, to a certain extent superfluous within the philosophy of anyone who truly understands the fundamental modes of action of this remarkable herb. It is, to a certain extent, inevitable that the fundamental changes which Aloe is capable of making within the body will help the body to fend off each and every chronic disease. Much though that may sound like a heresy to strictly orthodox clinicians, whose medical philosophy requires them to look at each and every labeled medical condition as though it were a separate entity, this author, who is himself so deeply rooted in medical science, now regards this as a truism. And that conclusion emanates from deep inquiry into the biochemical actions of Aloe at the cellular level. There is, indeed, every reason, through a process of scientific inference, to believe that each and every chronic disease will be found to respond to greater of lesser degree, to Aloe. The most likely exception to this is those genetic illnesses which are wholly determined by genetic error, but even with these there is a chance that the overall medical condition of the patient will be better for a certain toning up of cellular metabolism, such as Aloe can bring. This author's exploration of the literature has found a general absence of negative results when people have tried the use of Aloe against chronic disease. As has been shown, some of the papers on the subject report that 100% of patients responded to Aloe or very nearly so.

What are the limitations of Aloe? However remarkable, all medications have their limits. Genetically determined illness have just been mentioned. These include such rare, but wholly genetically determined illnesses as phenylketonuria, alcaptonuria, or porphyria, diseases which result from the genetic deletion of a single more or less essential enzyme. The much more common blood diseases of sickle cell anemia and thalassaemia similarly are determined by genetic error, and cannot expect any specific benefit from Aloe, though Aloe might conceivably help with some of their secondary problems. It should be born in mind, though, that in many other diseases which involve inherited factors, all that is inherited is a susceptibility, as in the case, for example, of Type 1 diabetes, the actual appearance of the disease being determined by other factors. In such diseases as these, Aloe may well have a real role to play.

Another limitation of Aloe is that it cannot be expected to fully protect people from those factors in the western lifestyle which lead towards chronic disease. What it can be expected to provide, from all the evidence given here, is a degree of protection against these things. Therefore, in this author's view, there will always be levels of cellular toxicity, arising from environmental poisons, from chemicals in processed foodstuffs etc., or arising from bacterial action in the bowel through poor diet, which Aloe cannot possibly be expected to counteract. There will also be levels of dietary deficiency, in respect of vitamins, essential fatty acids and, most especially, minerals, which cannot possibly be counteracted by the action of Aloe alone. Therefore, to get the best effect from the use of Aloe, it should always be accompanied by measures to ensure that the diet is also therapeutic and that, if the diet alone is not going to reliably provide more-than-adequate levels of vitamins, essential fatty acids and minerals, then supplements of these should also be used. The present author, being a practitioner of nutritional medicine, believes strongly that the above detailed aims should best be achieved by consulting a professional expert. This should always be a consideration wherever significant disease states exist. However, you need no practitioner whatsoever just to decide to use Aloe, which can be done by anyone following the guidelines given below.

Lastly among the limitations of Aloe, one has to be prepared to accept that some degrees of tissue damage brought about by some diseases, when they get to a certain point, are beyond repair by any means at all. Chronic diseases are, at their very worst, degenerative in character. Degeneration of tissues means that they die, and if they are replaced at all, they will tend to be replaced with connective tissue which will not perform the functions of the original tissues. The key factor in causing chronic disease is the accumulation of toxins, if you accept the naturopathic idiom. These toxins always have the potential to be removed by cleansing procedures. However, the longer the toxins remain in a tissue and the higher their concentration, the more damage and destruction will be wrought there. A long residence time for a high level of toxicity within tissues spells out the inevitability of toxic damage reaching the stage of degeneration. When this point is reached in the disease process, the question is not whether or not the toxins can be removed, because that is always likely to be possible with sufficiently strong naturopathic procedures, but to what extent the degenerative damage is capable of being repaired by the body afterwards. In such serious cases, Aloe is capable of giving a splendid boost to both cleansing and healing. The healing process equals repair. It is just that with very serious chronic ailments, it must always be recognized that some of this already-created damage will be impossible to repair. The advance of the disease may have been and should have been halted, and some repair of past damage may also be possible. Aloe can reasonably by expected to participate in quite a major way in these processes. However, some proportion of the already-inflicted damage is likely to prove irreparable. That proportion may be large or small depending upon the state of progression of the chronic ailment and the length of time for which it has been in place. That is, therefore a limitation of Aloe treatment, but it is also a limitation of all other treatment possibilities.

## Selection of the right Aloe Products

Any user of Aloe should bear in mind the recent history of Aloe, which is that whilst it has marvelous credentials as a curative herbal remedy, it has been much abused by the unscrupulous acts of certain suppliers. They have diluted the extracts with water and extended it dishonestly by the addition of inactive maltodextrin, dextrose or glycerol. It has also been subject to other forms of abuse which were not dishonest, but involved processing the plant in ways which failed, to various degrees, to preserve its biological activity. There are also operators who market only a distillate from Aloe. From what is known of the active ingredients of Aloe, there is absolutely no reason to expect that any significant amount of these will be present in such distillates. To all intents and purposes, these distillates must be virtually inactive in any biochemical sense, though whether or not they are capable of some homeopathic effect is entirely for speculation.

The biochemical control of Aloe quality is in its early days. It is not yet possible to directly monitor Aloe products for their content of active principles, since some of these are not yet sufficiently characterized.

However, The International Aloe Science Council has been able to set some standards, the application of which is certainly able to weed out the most obvious cases of abuse involving dilution, distillation or the addition of maltodextrin. The tests being applied at present are measurement of (1) calcium content (2) magnesium content (3) total solids content and (4) examination by a technique called high pressure liquid chromatography (HPLC) which shows up a peak which has become known as "E Peak" and consists of malic acid. None of these substances being measured here are the substances that are responsible for Aloe's biological actions, but they are criteria designed to weed out obvious fraud. So, this author's first recommendation to users is to check with the supplier whether the product comes from a manufacturer who has definitely had his products certified by The International Aloe Science Council. One should not be hesitant about asking this, nor should one be willing to accept fudged answers to this question, and if evidence of certification cannot be shown if asked, that is cause for suspicion.

In the UK it is possible to seek advice from the *Aloe vera* Information Service.

The next question concerns the selection between a whole leaf *Aloe vera* and a gel product. Most of the products on the market at present are products from the gel of the leaf. There is certainly nothing wrong with that and gel is the most long-established and longest recognized form of Aloe apart from the exudate, or "aloin" fraction, which is of a quite different nature. Previously, whole leaf Aloe extracts were not used because they would always have contained the "aloin" fraction, which was not wanted because of its purgative action, which would have been unwanted and unhelpful in a product being taken mainly for anti-inflammatory, immuno-stimulant and healing effects. The fact that Aloe leaf was composed of separate gel and rind provided a fortuitous way in which to furnish Aloe material which was virtually "aloin-free", simply by dissecting out the central gel section of the leaf. However, this fiddly dissection had to be hand done and was expensive, and discarding the rind was always an expensive option too, since the discarded rind undoubtedly contained further quantities of the same active principles which the gel contained, made unusable only by the presence of the "aloin". Recently the development of the technology required to produce a good quality whole leaf extract almost free from the purgative "aloin" components, has changed the picture, and certainly has changed the choice of options available to the user of Aloe. This technology has consisted of (a) the addition of cellulase enzyme to the disintegrated whole leaf prior to expressing the juice and (b) carbon filtration for efficient removal of the "aloin" fraction and so avoid making a product with an unwanted purgative action.

Whole leaf extract manufactured in this way contains a higher concentration of total solids than any gel extract. This is no surprise because the gel is a specialized water-storage tissue and one would expect its water content to be very high and its solids content very low. The whole leaf extract contains juice made from all the cells of the leaf, including the functional palisade layers and mesophyll layers of photosynthetic tissues, which have their place within the rind. Because these cell layers are highly active in metabolism they are bound to be rich in enzyme systems and all the other biochemicals which are prerequisites for an active metabolism. Any plant biochemist would therefore expect the content of soluble solids in the juice from these layers to be correspondingly much higher than in juice made solely from gel.

This proves to be the case in practice. The total solids level is from 1.6 to 3 times higher in the whole leaf extract than in the extract made just from gel. Total solids is one of the measures used by The International Aloe Science Council in assessing the genuineness of Aloe products. The others, as stated above, are calcium, magnesium and malic acid (E Peak). These parameters also are 1.6 to 3 times higher in the whole leaf extract than in the extract made just from gel. Although these measures are being made on substances which are not themselves among the active principles of Aloe, they have been adopted for the time being as official measures of the genuine nature of Aloe products. It is hard, therefore, to avoid the conclusion at this stage, that the whole leaf products are more concentrated than pure gel extracts and that they are therefore better also with regard to physiological activity.

This is where the subject rests at present, and it makes it necessary to recommend here that the best source of Aloe for most purposes will be the whole leaf extract.

There is little doubt that this subject will be investigated more fully in the coming years and more information about the direct measurement of the biological activities of whole leaf rxtract compared with the gel will be very welcome. As has been indicated already in chapter 2, detailed work to be done in the future is very likely to reveal that there are at least some important qualitative differences between the biological activities of whole leaf extract and gel. It is by no means impossible that gel will be shown to be prefewable in some particular applications.

Some unknowns relating to whole leaf extract have to do with the fact that the use of cellulase enzyme as a processing aid can affect the biological activity of the finished product. As to whether this is advantageous or not in the case of a particular product, depends upon the skill and knowledge of the manufacturer. It is also known that the carbon filtration stage, while being necessary, detracts to some degree from the potentially very high level of biological activity which whole leaf extracts could attain. So, managing the carbon filtration stage of manufacture so as to maximize the biological activity of the finished product will need to be a continuing pre-occupation of the manufacturers. It is certainly not feasible to skip the carbon-filtration to produce higher activity, since this would produce a poor-flavored product, and, through delivering an uncontrolled amount of "aloin" fraction, would be liable to give rise to purgative effects. We have seen in preceding chapters that some components of the "aloin" appear to be required for the fullest possible biological activity of Aloe, at least in certain of the specialized uses. Hence, fame and fortune may possibly await the manufacturer who chooses to sell a non-tasting capsule containing a distinctly sub-purgative dose of the "aloin" fraction, for use in conjunction with the taking of liquid *Aloe vera* products in serious medical applications.

## Dosage and Usage of Whole Leaf Extract

It should be noted here that manufacturers produce whole leaf extract (a) at its natural strength (b) at various levels of concentrate produced by evaporation - typically from twice the natural strength to ten times or more and (c) dried powders produced from whole leaf extract by evaporation followed by freeze-drying. Clearly all these products are active when manufacture is in good hands and the processes of evaporation and drying are conducted in ways sensitive to the known susceptibilities of the active ingredients of Aloe. This author considers that the natural strength of the product is too dilute for perfect convenience, but that the higher levels of concentration are likely to show some significant losses in activity in processing. Hence, moderate concentrates designated from 2X to 10X, and varying according to trade terminology and jargon 10X can be well recommended. Some products are likely to contain between 10,000 and 15,000mg per litre of methanol precipitable solids (MPS).

Dosage recommendations for this particular type of product would be from 25ml per day for routine precautionary use, 50ml per day for mildly therapeutic use and 100ml per day for stronger therapeutic applications. The product would be better taken one hour away from other food and drink (i.e. not eating or drinking for 1 hour either before or after the dose) and in the last two dose levels (therapeutic use) the daily dose should be divided between two half-doses per day, i.e., either 25ml twice per day or 50ml twice per day.

## Aloe Drinks

The above routine, using concentrates of pure Aloe, is recommended for anything from seriously intentioned preventive use right up to serious therapeutic application of Aloe vera. However, much Aloe vera is consumed in pleasantly fruit-flavoured drinks, where the user's intention is not so much to use Aloe vera for a medical purpose, but, rather, to enjoy a pleasant drink which will encompass some degree of beneficial effect. Such products have much to be said for them in this more light-hearted application. They may be based upon either the gel of whole leaf extract. Those which contain the gel may actually contain discernible pieces of solid gel material: This is likely to be good because such gel material has, inherently, not been disintegrated and altered in processing. Such products undoubtedly have a future too, for the organolepticcum social enjoyment of Aloe vera. These products also, should come from producers fully certified through The International Aloe Science Council.

## Topical Use

Finally, the application of Aloe to the skin, or to the accessible mucous membranes, via creams and ointments, has a long-standing role, both in home treatment and in hospital applications. These creams and ointments are readily available from manufacturers and their use for appropriate superficial conditions can be thoroughly recommended. However, these products also, should come from producers fully certified through The International Aloe Science Council who are prepared to showcopies of the certificates. Alternatively the 2X to 10X concentrates can be applied topically also using either cotton wool pad, or other means.

# SCIENTIFIC LITERATURE ON THE IMMUNOSTIMULANT ACTION OF ALOE

Davis RH, Parker WL, Sampson RT & Murdoch DP. "Isolation of a stimulatory system in an aloe extract." *J Am Podiatr Med Assoc* 81 (9); 473-478: 1991

Imanishi, K. "Aloctin A, an Active Substance of Aloe arborescens Miller as immunomodulator". 1993

Karaca, K., Sharma, J.M. & Nordgren, R. "Nitric Oxide production by chicken macrophages activated by Acemannan". *Int. J. Immuno Pharmacol.* 17(3); 183-8: 1995.

Pittman JC. "Immune enhancing effects of Aloe." Health Conscious 13 (1); 28-30: 1992.

Sheets, M.A. *et al.* "Studies on the effect of acemannan on retrovirus infections: clinical stabilization of feline virus-infected cats." *Mol. Biother.* 3; 41-45: 1991

Shida, T., Yagi, A., Nishimura, H., & Nishioka, I. "Effect of Aloe Extract on Peripheral Phagocytosis in Adult Bronchial Asthma". *Planta Med.* pp273-275: 1985

Solar S. *et al.* "Mise en evidence et etude proprietes immuno-stimulantes díun extrait isole et partiellement purifie a partir díaloe vahombe". *Archives de l'Institut Pasteur de Madagascar* 47; 9-39: 1979.

't Hart LA, Nibbering PH, Van Den Barselaar MT, Van Dijk H, Van Den Berg AJ & Labadie RP. "Effects of low molecular constituents from aloe vera gel on oxidative metabolism and cytotoxic and bacterial activities of human neutrophils." *Int J Immuno-pharmacol* 12 (4); 427-434: 1990

't Hart LA, Van Den Berg AJ, Klus L, Van Dijk & Labadle RP. "An anti-complementary polysaccharide with immunological adjuvant activity from the leaf parenchyma gel of Aloe vera." *Planta Med* 55 (6); 509-12: 1989.

't Hart LA, Van Enckevort PH, Van Dijk H, Zaat R & De Silva KT. "Two functionally and chemically distinct immuno-modulatory compounds in the gel of Aloe vera." *J Ethnopharmacol* May-Jun 23 (1); 61-71: 1988

Winters, W.D. "Immunoreactive Lectins in Leaf Gel from Aloe barbadensis Miller." *Phytotherapy Res.* 7; 523-525: 1993

Womble, D. & Helderman, J.H. "Enhancement of Allo-Responsiveness of Human Lymphocytes by Acemannan (Carrisyn)." *Int. J. Immuno-pharmacol.* 10(8); 967-974: 1988

Yagi, A. "Effect of Amino Acids in Aloe Extract on Phagocytosis by peripheral neutrophils in Adult Bronchial Asthma." *Jpn J. Allergol.* 36 (12); 1094-1101: 1987

# Index

calcium receptors 63
California, southern 6
campesterol 43, 99
cancer 8, 48, 53, 93, 94
*Candida albicans* infection 8, 32, 47
carbon dioxide 11
carbon treatment 26
carbuncles 8
cardiac glycoside 19
Caribbean 6
cascara (*Rhamnus purshiana*) 32
catabolic 109
cell constituents 10, 55, 56, 60, 65
cells, red blood 59, 70
cellular responses 64
cellulase 26
cellulose fibers 12, 25
Cera 86
chemical energy 10
chemotaxis 71
cholecystokinin 51
cholesterol 56, 59, 99
chromatography 45
Chronic Fatigue Syndrome 8, 82
chronic diseases 18
chrysophanol glucoside 31
chysophanol 31
*Cinchona* 20
citric acid cycle 40
citric 22
Cohen 106
colds 8
colic 8
colitis 16, 51
Collins 86
complex carbohydrate 79
compositional changes 24
connective tissues 17, 103
constancy of internal environment 67
constipation 8, 32
corrosive chemicals 16
cow's milk 113
creams 122
Crewe 86, 87
Crohn's disease 16, 113
cuticle 11

cysteine 39
cytosol 57
dandruff 8

Davis 81, 85, 95, 98, 99, 102, 103, 106
de-aloinized whole leaf extract 37, 48
dentistry 47, 50, 97
dermatitis in dogs 87
dermatitis 8, 86
dermatoses 86
detoxification 18
diabetes (Type I) 8, 47, 51, 75, 87, 89,
103, 112, 116
diabetes (Type II) 105
dialysis 45
diarrhea 89
Didonato, 103
DieGelmann 106
digestive system 47, 48, 82, 91
digitalis 19, 20, 30
Dioscoroides 4
disinfectant agent 48
DNA 57, 59, 103
dosage 121
drug steroids 30
drying operation 28
duodenal cap lesions 90
duodenal ulcers 8
dynamic equilibrium 59
edema 8, 92
efficacy 6, 8
Egypt's "Papyrus Embers" 4
emodin 34
energy 55
enzyme 25
eosinophils 73
epidermis 11
Epstein-Barr virus 82
essential fatty acids 117
evaporation 27
extract 27
exudate 12, 14, 15, 29, 32, 33, 35

Farida 89
fatty acids 11, 59

125

insect bites 8
insects 19
insoluble matter 26
insomnia 8
insulin 51, 60, 88, 109
insulitis 112
interferon 71, 72
interleukin-1 108
International Aloe Science Council
118, 120, 122
intestinal bacteria 110
intestines 39
Islets of Langerhans 72, 112
isoanthorin 31
isobarbaloin 31
isoeleutherol glucoside 31

Japanese research 90
jelly-fish stings 8
joints 78

Kaplan 106
keratin 11
kidney tubule cells 59
kidneys 75
kinins 71
*Klebsiella pneumoniae* 49, 79
Krebs cycle 40
Kupffer cells 72
Kuwait 89
laxative 14, 32
"leaky" gut 92
lectin activity 45
leg ulcers 86
leukocytes 71
leukotrienes 71, 72
Levenstein 85
light absorption 12
Lily family 1
liver 75
lucerne 38
lumen 58
lupeol 99
lupus erythematosus 75
lymphatic system 67, 69, 72, 111

lymphocytes 59, 73, 74, 76, 77
lymphoid tissue 69, 70
lysosome 58, 72

macrophages 59, 72, 80, 102, 106
magnesium 41, 42, 90, 110, 118
magnesium lactate 40, 90
malic acid 22, 118, 120
maltodextrin 118
mannan 45, 108
mannose 38, 44, 45, 46, 80, 81, 102
   -6-phosphate 102
   -containing glycoproteins 102
mast cells 73
medicine 26
menstrual cramps 8
menstrual flow 14
methanol precipitable solids (MPS)
21, 22, 44, 121
methyl alcohol 21
minerals 10, 38, 40, 41, 117
mitochondria 58
mitogenic effect 108
mobile protein carrier 61
mucopolysaccharides 21
multiple sclerosis 112
muscle cells 59
muscle spasms 105

N-acetyl glucosamine 80
naturopathic philosophy 110
nausea 8
nerve cells 59
neutrophils 72, 77, 80
New World 6
nitric oxide 79
non-insulin-dependent diabetes 88
nondialysable material 45
North America 6

ointments 122
opiate receptors 63
organelles 57, 58
organic acids 38, 39, 40
otolaryngology 48, 52, 97